INFORMING SOCIAL SECURITY'S PROCESS FOR

Financial Capability Determination

Committee to Evaluate the Social Security Administration's Capability Determination Process for Adult Beneficiaries

Paul S. Appelbaum, Carol Mason Spicer, Frank R. Valliere, *Editors*

Board on the Health of Select Populations

Institute of Medicine

The National Academies of
SCIENCES · ENGINEERING · MEDICINE

THE NATIONAL ACADEMIES PRESS
Washington, DC
www.nap.edu

THE NATIONAL ACADEMIES PRESS 500 Fifth Street, NW Washington, DC 20001

This activity was supported by Contract No. SS00-13-60048-0005 with the U.S. Social Security Administration. Any opinions, findings, conclusions, or recommendations expressed in this publication do not necessarily reflect the views of any organization or agency that provided support for the project.

International Standard Book Number-13: 978-0-309-39257-0
International Standard Book Number-10: 0-309-39257-8
Digital Object Identifier: 10.17226/21922

Additional copies of this report are available for sale from the National Academies Press, 500 Fifth Street, NW, Keck 360, Washington, DC 20001; (800) 624-6242 or (202) 334-3313; http://www.nap.edu.

Printed in the United States of America

Suggested citation: National Academies of Sciences, Engineering, and Medicine. 2016. *Informing Social Security's process for financial capability determination.* Washington, DC: The National Academies Press. doi: 10.17226/21922.

The National Academies of

SCIENCES · ENGINEERING · MEDICINE

The **National Academy of Sciences** was established in 1863 by an Act of Congress, signed by President Lincoln, as a private, nongovernmental institution to advise the nation on issues related to science and technology. Members are elected by their peers for outstanding contributions to research. Dr. Ralph J. Cicerone is president.

The **National Academy of Engineering** was established in 1964 under the charter of the National Academy of Sciences to bring the practices of engineering to advising the nation. Members are elected by their peers for extraordinary contributions to engineering. Dr. C. D. Mote, Jr., is president.

The **National Academy of Medicine** (formerly the Institute of Medicine) was established in 1970 under the charter of the National Academy of Sciences to advise the nation on medical and health issues. Members are elected by their peers for distinguished contributions to medicine and health. Dr. Victor J. Dzau is president.

The three Academies work together as the **National Academies of Sciences, Engineering, and Medicine** to provide independent, objective analysis and advice to the nation and conduct other activities to solve complex problems and inform public policy decisions. The Academies also encourage education and research, recognize outstanding contributions to knowledge, and increase public understanding in matters of science, engineering, and medicine.

Learn more about the National Academies of Sciences, Engineering, and Medicine at **www.national-academies.org**.

COMMITTEE TO EVALUATE THE SOCIAL SECURITY ADMINISTRATION'S CAPABILITY DETERMINATION PROCESS FOR ADULT BENEFICIARIES

PAUL S. APPELBAUM (*Chair*), Elizabeth Dollard Professor of Psychiatry, Medicine and Law, and Director, Division of Law, Ethics and Psychiatry, Department of Psychiatry, Columbia University

KAREN E. ANDERSON, Director, Huntington Disease Care, Education and Research Center, and Associate Professor of Psychiatry and Neurology, Georgetown University Medical Center and MedStar Georgetown University Hospital

MARÍA P. ARANDA, Associate Professor, University of Southern California School of Social Work

NANCY BAGATELL, Associate Professor, Division of Occupational Science and Occupational Therapy, University of North Carolina at Chapel Hill

JULIE BIRKENMAIER, Professor, Saint Louis University School of Social Work

NANCY N. DUBLER, Professor Emerita, Albert Einstein College of Medicine; Consultant for Ethics, New York City Health and Hospital Corporation; and Adjunct Professor, Division of Medical Ethics, New York University Langone Medical Center

LAURA B. DUNN, Director, Geriatric Psychiatry Fellowship Training Program and Professor, Department of Psychiatry and Behavioral Sciences, Stanford University

ALAN M. JETTE, Professor of Health Policy & Management, Boston University School of Public Health

DAVID A. LOEWENSTEIN, Director and Professor of Neuropsychology, Department of Psychiatry and Behavioral Sciences, University of Miami Miller School of Medicine

MARC A. NORMAN, Professor, Medical Neuropsychology, and Director, Neuropsychiatry/Epilepsy Clinical Evaluation Program, University of California, San Diego

ELDAR SHAFIR, William Stewart Tod Professor of Psychology and Public Affairs, Department of Psychology and the Woodrow Wilson School of Public and International Affairs, Princeton University

KELLY A. THOMPSON, Thompson Wildhack PLC, Arlington, Virginia

Consultant

ALLEN W. HEINEMANN, Director, Center for Rehabilitation Outcomes Research, Rehabilitation Institute of Chicago

IOM Fellow

KENDALL M. CAMPBELL, Co-Director, Center for Underrepresented Minorities in Academic Medicine, and Associate Professor, Family Medicine and Rural Health, Florida State University College of Medicine

IOM Project Staff

CAROL MASON SPICER, Study Director
FRANK R. VALLIERE, Associate Program Officer
JENNIFER FLAUBERT, Associate Program Officer (since December 2015)
NICOLE GORMLEY, Senior Program Assistant
PAMELA RAMEY-McCRAY, Administrative Assistant
FREDERICK ERDTMANN, Director, Board on the Health of Select Populations

Reviewers

This report has been reviewed in draft form by individuals chosen for their diverse perspectives and technical expertise. The purpose of this independent review is to provide candid and critical comments that will assist the institution in making its published report as sound as possible and to ensure that the report meets institutional standards for objectivity, evidence, and responsiveness to the study charge. The review comments and draft manuscript remain confidential to protect the integrity of the deliberative process. We wish to thank the following individuals for their review of this report:

Henry Aaron, The Brookings Institution
Sara S. Bachman, Boston University School of Social Work
Denise Burnette, Columbia University School of Social Work
Lisa Dixon, Columbia University Medical Center
Kathryn Edin, Johns Hopkins University
Eric B. Elbogen, University of North Carolina at Chapel Hill School of Medicine
Jason Karlawish, University of Pennsylvania
Kristi L. Kirschner, University of Illinois at Chicago
Daniel C. Marson, The University of Alabama at Birmingham
Barton W. Palmer, University of California, San Diego
Elizabeth K. Rasch, National Institutes of Health
Marc I. Rosen, Yale University School of Medicine
Elyn Saks, University of Southern California Gould School of Law

Although the reviewers listed above provided many constructive comments and suggestions, they were not asked to endorse the report's conclusions or recommendations, nor did they see the final draft of the report before its release. The review of this report was overseen by **Georges Benjamin,** American Public Health Association, and **Bradford H. Gray,** The Urban Institute. They were responsible for making certain that an independent examination of this report was carried out in accordance with institutional procedures and that all review comments were carefully considered. Responsibility for the final content of this report rests entirely with the authoring committee and the institution.

Preface

The U.S. Social Security Administration (SSA) provides benefits to disabled adults and children, offering vital financial support to more than 17 million disabled Americans. Of that group, approximately 5 million have been deemed—by virtue of youth or mental or physical impairment—incapable of managing or directing the management of their benefits.[1] Hence, a representative payee has been appointed to receive and disburse SSA payments for these beneficiaries to ensure that their basic needs for shelter, food, and clothing arc met. Periodically, however, concerns have been expressed about the accuracy of the process by which SSA determines whether beneficiaries are capable of managing their benefits, with some evidence suggesting that underdetection of incapable recipients may be a particular problem.

The importance of creating as accurate a process as possible for incapability determinations is underscored by the consequences of incorrectly identifying recipients either as incapable when they can manage their benefits or as capable when they cannot. Given the importance of individual autonomy in decision making in a democratic society, deprivation of the right to manage one's money—which ensues from a finding of incapability—represents a serious infringement on liberty that should occur only when absolutely necessary. Conversely, failure to identify beneficiaries who are incapable of managing their funds means abandoning a vulnerable population to potential homelessness, hunger, and disease. Needless to say, neither error is desirable.

[1] The prepublication version of this report erroneously included a group of nondisabled beneficiaries in the numbers provided in the preceding sentences. These numbers were revised for accuracy.

With support from SSA, the Institute of Medicine (IOM) of the National Academies of Sciences, Engineering, and Medicine convened a committee to evaluate SSA's capability determination process. In pursuit of that goal, the committee reviewed the relevant professional literatures in several languages, heard testimony from researchers who study the capability determination process and from persons directly involved with it, considered existing assessment tools and their applicability to this process, looked at comparable programs in the public and private sectors in Canada and the United States, and obtained background information and data from SSA on the operation of its system.

Drawing on all of these sources, the committee formulated a number of conclusions and recommendations that it believes can inform and guide efforts to improve the current capability determination process. Most notably, the committee concluded that basing capability determinations on evidence of beneficiaries' actual performance in meeting their basic needs is superior to office-based assessment of individuals' financial competence. In such a performance-based process, priority is given to information from persons who are in direct contact with beneficiaries and are in a position to know about their financial performance.

On behalf of the committee, I want to thank all of the individuals who shared their time and expertise during the committee's information-gathering sessions. Special thanks go to Winthrop Cashdollar at America's Health Insurance Plans for collecting and compiling information from a number of private companies that provide disability income protection coverage about their procedures for determining when a claimant is not competent to handle disability income benefits. I also extend thanks to the IOM staff members who played a key role in the production of this report, including Rick Erdtmann (board director), Carol Mason Spicer (study director), Frank Valliere (associate program officer), Nicole Gormley (senior program assistant), and Julie Wiltshire (financial associate). Research assistance was provided by Daniel Bearss and Rebecca Morgan. Rona Briere and Alisa Decatur are to be credited for the superb editorial assistance they provided in preparing the final report.

Finally, as committee chair, I want to express my appreciation for the hard work and collegial approaches of all the committee members. I know they share my hope that this report can have a positive impact on the lives of persons with disabilities who may need assistance in managing their benefits.

Paul S. Appelbaum, *Chair*
Committee to Evaluate the Social Security
Administration's Capability Determination
Process for Adult Beneficiaries

Contents

APPENDIXES

Boxes, Figures, and Tables

BOXES

FIGURES

TABLES

Acronyms and Abbreviations

ACED	Assessment of Capacity for Everyday Decision-making
ADA	Americans with Disabilities Act
AHIP	America's Health Insurance Plans
ASD	autism spectrum disorder
ATM	automated teller machine
CAFI	Clinician Assessment of Financial Incapability
CDR	continuing disability review
CPP	Canada Pension Plan
CSRS	Civil Service Retirement System
DDS	Disability Determination Services
DE	disability examiner
DEBT	Disability Examiner Basic Training Program
DI	Disability Insurance
DSM-IV	*Diagnostic and Statistical Manual of Mental Disorders, Fourth Edition*
EFB	Everyday Functioning Battery
ESDC	Employment and Social Development Canada
FCAI	Financial Competence Assessment Instrument
FCI	Financial Capacity Instrument
FCI-SF	Financial Capacity Instrument-Short Form
FEGLI	Federal Employees' Group Life Insurance

FEHB	Federal Employee Health Benefits
FERS	Federal Employee Retirement System
FISCAL	Financial Incapability Structured Clinical Assessment done Longitudinally
HRSA	Health Resources and Services Administration
IADL	instrumental activity of daily living
ICD	*International Classification of Diseases*
ICF	*International Classification of Functioning, Disability and Health*
ILS	Independent Living Scales
ILSS	Independent Living Skills Survey
IOM	Institute of Medicine
KELS	Kohlman Evaluation of Living Skills
MMM	Money Mismanagement Measure
NADE	National Association of Disability Examiners
NCE	National Counselor Examination
NICS	National Instant Criminal Background Check System
NPV	negative predictive value
OAS	Old Age Security
OASDI	Old-Age, Survivors, and Disability Insurance
OASI	Old-Age and Survivors Insurance
OIDAP	Occupational Information Development Advisory Panel (SSA)
OIG	Office of the Inspector General
OIG-SSA	Office of the Inspector General for the Social Security Administration
OPM	U.S. Office of Personnel Management
POA	power of attorney
POMS	Program Operations Manual System
PPV	positive predictive value
RVSR	Rating Veterans Service Representative
SES	socioeconomic status
SGA	substantial gainful activity
SLOF	Specific Levels of Function
SSA	U.S. Social Security Administration

SSDI	Social Security Disability Insurance
SSI	Supplemental Security Income
THRIFT	Timeline Historical Review of Income and Financial Transactions
VA	U.S. Department of Veterans Affairs
VBA	Veterans Benefits Administration
VSCM	Veterans Service Center Manager
VSR	Veterans Service Representative
WHO	World Health Organization

Summary[1]

The U.S. Social Security Administration (SSA) administers the Old-Age, Survivors, and Disability Insurance (OASDI) and Supplemental Security Income (SSI) programs, providing benefits to approximately 64 million Americans. Within OASDI, Old-Age and Survivors Insurance (OASI) pays benefits to retired workers who have paid into the program and their dependents and survivors, while Social Security Disability Insurance (SSDI) provides benefits to adults with disabilities who have worked and paid into the Disability Insurance trust fund and to their spouses and adult children who are unable to work because of disability.[2] SSI, a means-tested program based on income and financial assets, provides income assistance from U.S. Treasury general funds to adults aged 65 or older, individuals who are blind, and disabled adults and children. As of December 2014, approximately 48 million individuals received OASI benefits, about 11 million received SSDI benefits, and about 8 million received assistance through the SSI program. Of the roughly 64 million beneficiaries, approximately 3 million received benefits through both OASDI and SSI.

The Social Security Act Amendments of 1939 authorized the Commissioner of Social Security to make benefit payments to an individual

---

[1] This summary does not include references. Citations to support the text, conclusions, and recommendations herein are provided in the body of the report.

[2] Disabled beneficiaries who are now adults but became disabled prior to age 22, which SSA refers to as *disabled adult child beneficiaries*, receive benefits based on their parents' Social Security earnings record. To be eligible for disabled widow(er) benefits, the widow(er) must be between the ages of 50 and 59, prove his or her relationship to the disabled worker, and demonstrate his or her disability.

or organization other than the beneficiary when doing so would serve the beneficiary's interest. SSA uses the term *capability* to denote the ability of beneficiaries to manage or direct the management of their SSA benefits. SSA presumes that adult beneficiaries are capable unless there is evidence to the contrary. If there is some question as to whether a beneficiary's mental or physical impairments prevent that individual from managing or directing the management of his or her benefits, SSA makes a determination regarding the beneficiary's capability. If SSA determines that a beneficiary is incapable, the agency assigns a representative payee to receive and manage the beneficiary's benefits. The representative payee must use the benefits in the beneficiary's interest, although he or she may distribute small portions of the payment directly to the beneficiary.[3] The main goal of representative payment is to ensure that the beneficiary's interests are being met. Recognizing the importance of the representative payee program to the well-being of beneficiaries in need, SSA often has sought to improve various aspects of the program, conducting internal reviews and seeking expert advice from external sources. Although the process for determining whether a beneficiary is capable has received some attention, much of the focus of these past efforts has been on the performance of the representative payees assigned to those beneficiaries determined to be incapable.

As part of a full review of the representative payee program, SSA asked the Institute of Medicine (IOM) of the National Academies of Sciences, Engineering, and Medicine to convene a committee with relevant expertise to evaluate SSA's capability determination process for adult beneficiaries and provide recommendations for improving the accuracy and efficiency of the agency's policy and procedures for making these determinations (see Box S-1 for the committee's statement of task). In carrying out this task, the committee was asked to address topics including capability determination processes used in at least three similar benefit programs, requisite abilities for managing or directing the management of benefits, methods and measures for assessing capability, the use of capacity assessment tools, appropriate roles for SSA and state Disability Determination Services employees, and effects on the beneficiary of appointing a representative payee. To address this task, the IOM convened a 12-member committee that included experts in the areas of psychology, neuropsychology, psychiatry, social work, occupational therapy and rehabilitation, behavioral economics, bioethics, and law (see Appendix D for biographical sketches of the committee members).

At the committee's first meeting, SSA representatives clarified that the committee should focus on adults with disabilities. Although much of the information developed in the present report is applicable to all types

[3] This sentence was modified from the prepublication version of the report.

BOX S-1
Statement of Task

An ad hoc committee will conduct a study to evaluate the U.S. Social Security Administration's (SSA's) capability determination process for adult beneficiaries. In carrying out this task, the committee will

1. Familiarize itself with SSA's current policy and procedures for capability determinations for adult beneficiaries;
2. Provide an overview of the capability determination processes in at least three similar benefit programs (at least one government program and one private-sector program);
3. Compare SSA's program to these other programs; and
4. Provide recommendations to improve the accuracy and efficiency of SSA's policy and procedures for capability determinations.

To accomplish these objectives, the committee shall consider the following topics:

1. Capability determination processes used by other similar benefit programs;
2. Abilities required to manage, and direct the management of, benefits;
3. Effective methods and measures for assessing capability;
4. Use of capacity assessments tools;
5. Appropriate roles of SSA employees, state Disability Determination Services employees, and others in making capability determinations; and
6. Effects of SSA's decision to appoint a payee on the beneficiary.

of beneficiaries, issues unique to retirement beneficiaries and to the transition from child beneficiary to adult beneficiary are outside the scope of this study.

At its open meeting sessions, the committee heard presentations from representatives of SSA, the National Association of Disability Examiners, other benefit programs, and stakeholder organizations. Presentations also were made by experts in the assessment of financial capability, the impacts of the representative payee system on beneficiaries, the abilities needed to manage or direct the management of benefits, and the effects of everyday surroundings and stressors on an individual's capability (see Appendix A for the open session agendas). The committee's extensive literature review included reports of the Office of the Inspector General for SSA (OIG-SSA) and the Representative Payment Advisory Committee, as well as previous IOM and National Research Council reports relevant to the topic.

CAPABILITY DETERMINATION IN NON-SSA BENEFIT PROGRAMS

The committee compared SSA's capability determination process with those of the U.S. Department of Veterans Affairs (VA), the U.S. Office of Personnel Management (OPM), and Service Canada's Canada Pension Plan (CPP) and Old Age Security programs. In addition, with America's Health Insurance Plans (AHIP)[4] acting as an intermediary, the committee received information compiled from five private disability income protection insurers regarding their approaches to determining capability.

All of the programs reviewed focus on some combination of legal, medical, and lay evidence[5] in determining whether a beneficiary needs a representative payee, although the type of evidence emphasized varies across programs. For example, SSA considers medical evidence but requires lay evidence of incapability in making a determination. The VA and Service Canada require evidence from a medical professional, and OPM requires information from both a medical provider and two sources familiar with the beneficiary. SSA, OPM, Service Canada, and private insurers accept legal evidence of incompetency as sufficient evidence of incapability, while the VA does not consider legal evidence, such as a court decree of incompetency, to be binding.

The committee found no gold standard for determining financial capability among the programs it reviewed. Nonetheless, each program has unique aspects that the committee considers good practice and that, taken together, can contribute to a more procedurally sound process. These include SSA's and OPM's requirement for lay evidence to find a beneficiary incapable, which provides the opportunity to obtain information about beneficiaries' real-world financial performance; the VA's supervised direct payment option for individuals who are determined incompetent but able to manage their benefits with supervision, which reflects a model of supported decision making; and OPM's instructions to individuals providing evidence to inform capability determinations.

EFFECTS OF APPOINTMENT OF REPRESENTATIVE PAYEES ON BENEFICIARIES

Representative payee programs have been found to have significant and positive effects on a beneficiary's ability to live independently, which

[4] AHIP is the national trade association representing the health insurance industry.

[5] SSA defines "lay evidence" as anything other than legal or medical evidence. It can be provided by anyone with direct knowledge of facts or circumstances regarding the beneficiary in his or her daily life; this may include nonprofessionals (e.g., relatives, friends, neighbors) and health and social service professionals (e.g., social workers, occupational therapists, rehabilitation specialists, adult protective services workers).

in turn affects the individual's health and well-being. Appointment of representative payees is associated with increased ability to meet basic needs; declines in homelessness, victimization, and arrests; fewer hospitalizations; and improved substance abuse outcomes. Although research results are mixed as to whether the representative payee arrangement actually reduces substance abuse, clients with representative payees are more likely to stay engaged in treatment.

Despite such positive effects, appointment of a representative payee also has potential negative consequences. SSA representative payees are most commonly friends or family members of the beneficiaries. Such an arrangement can have significant negative effects on beneficiaries' relationships with those serving in this role; for example, beneficiaries can be negatively affected by strain in their familial relationships resulting from conflict over the money management responsibilities of family members acting as representative payees. In addition, being able to control how one's money is spent is considered an essential element of self-determination and for many is critical to feelings of self-worth. Loss of control over finances can provoke fear and anxiety, be seen as a threat to autonomy, and encourage dependence. In addition, having a representative payee may be perceived as stigmatizing.

Ultimately, the decision to appoint a representative payee entails weighing the beneficiary's personal autonomy and preferences against interventions that, while infringing on the beneficiary's autonomy, are meant to protect his or her best interests. Errors in either direction can have substantial negative effects on beneficiaries. To deem someone incapable when he or she is not erodes personal liberty, creates stigma through labeling, leaves the individual open to exploitation, and deprives the person of the freedom to direct personally appropriate actions based on long-held values and preferences. On the other hand, permitting someone who is not financially capable to continue to manage personal financial affairs may cause the person preventable harm as a result of the mismanagement of funds and an increased potential for victimization by others.

FINANCIAL CAPABILITY

SSA defines (financial) *capability* as a beneficiary's ability to *manage* or *direct the management of* his or her benefits. In keeping with the goal of ensuring that a beneficiary's interests are met, the committee understands *financial capability* as involving the management or direction of the management of one's funds in a way that routinely meets one's best interests. Consistent with SSA's guidance to employees and representative payees, the committee interprets meeting one's best interests as routinely[6] satisfying the basic needs of food, shelter, and clothing—a standard that is minimally restrictive of the liberty of beneficiaries to manage their own affairs.

In evaluating financial capability, the committee distinguishes between *financial performance* and *financial competence* (see Figure S-1). It defines *financial performance* as an individual's degree of success in handling financial demands in the context of the stresses, supports, contextual cues, and resources in his or her actual environment. *Financial competence* refers to the financial skills one possesses, as demonstrated through *financial knowledge* and *financial judgment*, typically assessed in a controlled (e.g., office or other clinical) setting.

Financial knowledge is possession of the declarative knowledge (i.e., information that a person knows) and procedural knowledge (i.e., knowing how to perform a task) required to manage one's finances (e.g., the concept of money, values of currency, making change, check writing, use of automatic teller machines, and online banking procedures). *Financial judgment* is possession of the abilities (understanding, reasoning, and appreciation) needed to make financial decisions and choices that serve the individual's best interests.

An individual may be financially competent in an office or clinical setting but may not exercise his or her financial knowledge and judgment in a real-life setting sufficiently to meet his or her basic needs. Conversely, an individual may fail to demonstrate financial knowledge or judgment in a controlled setting but may perform effectively with the assistance of support systems in his or her environment. Because contextual factors can enhance or diminish individuals' (real-world) financial performance relative to what would be expected based on the financial competence they exhibit in controlled settings, it is important to consider more than financial competence when thinking about financial capability.

Successful financial performance reflects sufficient financial competence (knowledge and judgment) to implement financial decisions in the real world, that is, the presence of sufficient cognitive, perceptual, affective, communicative, and interpersonal abilities to manage or direct others to manage one's benefits. For this reason, the committee concludes that evidence of beneficiaries' real-world financial performance in meeting their basic needs is the best indicator of their financial capability. Preference for financial performance in determining financial capability is consistent

[6] The committee recognizes that circumstances and personal preferences at times may require or lead individuals to forgo a basic need, such as food. Nevertheless, individuals' overall behavior may still reflect an ability to use their benefits to meet their basic needs over time. When that occurs, their needs are being met routinely, in the sense in which that term is used in this report.

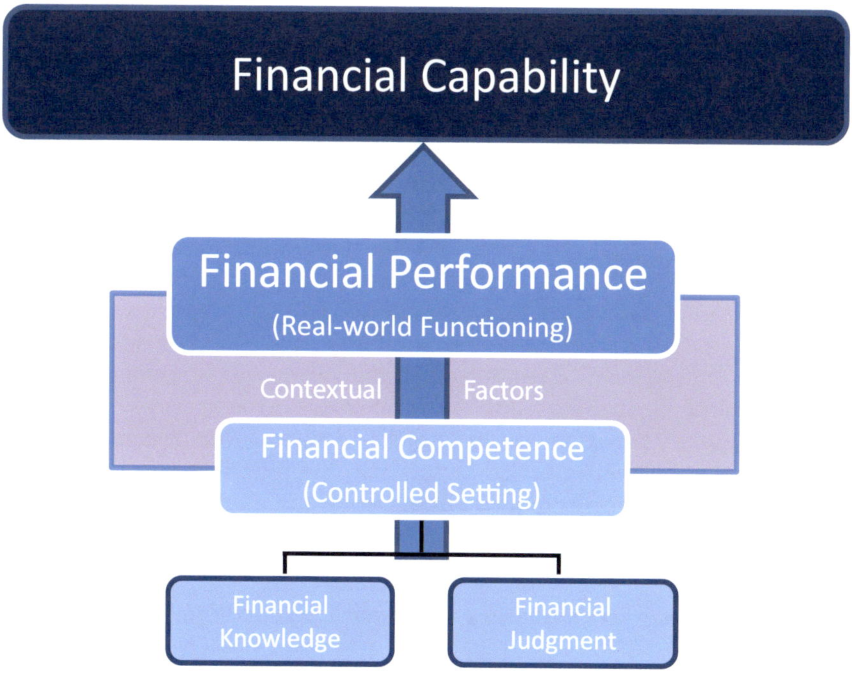

FIGURE S-1 Conceptual model of financial capability.

both with the movement toward conceptualizing disability in terms of the interaction between an individual's environment and his or her functional capacity and with the reform of guardianship laws during the past 25 years.

MENTAL AND PHYSICAL DISORDERS THAT MAY AFFECT FINANCIAL CAPABILITY

The presence of certain cognitive disorders, such as a well-documented history of severe intellectual disability or advanced Alzheimer's disease, may be sufficient for a determination of incapability, but such examples are few in number.

Disorders with Cognitive Effects

Evaluation of financial capability is important for individuals with disorders severe enough to lead to work-related disability that negatively affect the cognitive domains relevant to financial competence (e.g., general cognitive/intellectual ability, attention and vigilance, learning and memory, executive function, social cognition, language and communication). The challenge is that while the presence of such disorders increases the need for assessment of financial capability, ordinarily neither a diagnosis nor medical evidence alone is sufficient for making a capability determination.

One difficulty is the variable impact of disorders on the individuals affected; different people experience and respond to medical conditions differently. Another difficulty is the lack of correlation in many cases between the severity of clinical symptoms and functional limitations. Furthermore, the impairment severity threshold for determining work-related disability may reasonably differ from that required to justify interference with beneficiaries' autonomy in managing their disability payments. For this reason, it would be imprudent to attempt to map the level of impairment associated with financial incapability onto the level of impairment for work-related disability, such as that contained in SSA's *Listing of Impairments*. Finally, as noted above, environmental factors may support continued successful financial performance in individuals experiencing a level of cognitive impairment sufficient to qualify for SSA disability benefits.

Disorders with No or Minimal Cognitive Effects

Individuals with certain physical impairments may require assistance to accomplish the physical tasks entailed in managing their benefits, but in the absence of cognitive impairment, they retain the ability to direct others to manage their benefits. They therefore are financially capable. Rare exceptions to this observation are physical impairments that completely preclude communication with others to direct the management of benefits even with the use of assistive communication devices—for example, myopathies (e.g., mitochondrial myopathies) and neuromuscular disorders (e.g., advanced ALS [amyotrophic lateral sclerosis] or locked-in syndrome) of such severity that any form of communication has become impossible.

ASSESSMENT OF FINANCIAL COMPETENCE AND PERFORMANCE

Assessment Instruments

The committee reviewed various instruments used to assess different components of financial capability (i.e., financial capacity, financial judgment, financial performance). In principle, such instruments could be helpful to medical and other professionals in gathering evidence of beneficiaries' financial performance. However, many of the instruments identified by the committee are designed to assess financial competence in an office or clinical setting. Some of the instruments appear to measure financial performance in a real-world setting, but most of them rely primarily on self-reported behavior. This is a limitation in that information provided by the individual being assessed may reflect that person's lack of awareness of his or her impairment or deliberate efforts to conceal it. While some of these instruments show good psychometric properties in relation to other assessment methods, sufficient data on reliability and validity across populations are not yet available to warrant recommending their routine use.

Sources of Evidence

Financial performance in real-world situations can best be captured by those professionals and others who have first-hand knowledge of and experience with how an individual functions in his or her environment and who have sufficient opportunities to observe the individual in that environment over an extended period of time. Reliable first-hand or collateral information regarding an individual's real-world financial performance is particularly helpful, because, as noted above, information provided by the individual being assessed may reflect that person's lack of awareness of his or her impairment or deliberate efforts to conceal it. However, the reliability of information provided by third-party informants varies as well. Some informants lack the opportunity to observe financial performance, while others spend insufficient time with the individual to assess his or her performance accurately. Informants also may under- or overestimate an individual's financial abilities for a variety of reasons. A relative might underestimate or underreport an individual's financial abilities in the hope of gaining access to the person's funds or overestimate an individual's abilities so as not to alienate the person.

RECOMMENDATIONS

Evidence for Determining Financial Capability

SSA's requirement for "lay" evidence of beneficiaries' financial performance in making capability determinations is consistent with the committee's conclusion that evidence of real-world financial performance is the most reliable basis for making such determinations. As noted, however, the reliability of third-party informants varies. In addition, most informants, including professionals, are not trained specifically in assessment of financial performance and competence and would benefit from detailed direction as to the type of information that is helpful to SSA in making capability determinations. Currently, SSA provides little formal guidance to medical professionals and no formal guidance to other informants. The committee therefore makes the following recommendation:

Recommendation 1. The U.S. Social Security Administration (SSA) should provide detailed guidance to professional and lay informants regarding the information it would find most helpful for making capability determinations, including (1) information about specific aspects of beneficiaries' financial performance in meeting their basic needs and, when information about performance is unavailable, about their financial competence; and (2) information that would enable SSA to judge the validity of the evidence provided by the informant.

With respect to financial performance, SSA's guidance to all informants could be based on the questions it currently provides to field officers. There are times when no or very limited information is available about a beneficiary's financial performance—for example, when the person has had no funds to manage or when no third-party informant with knowledge of the person's performance can be identified. In such cases, evidence of financial competence may need to be used to inform capability determinations. Guidance pertaining to financial competence could include questions such as those developed by CPP along with requests that the basis for informants' answers be specified.

To enable SSA to judge the validity of information from informants, it is important that evidence provided for capability determinations specify how well and for how long the informant has known the individual and the nature of their relationship.[7] It is also important to specify the extent to which (1) the informant's judgment is based on observed behavior; (2) the informant's judgment is based on the individual's self-report; (3) the informant's judgment is based on information from collateral informants, and the perceived quality of these informants; and (4) in the case of professionals, the judgment is based on the individual's medical record and the assessments of other health care professionals (including other physicians, psychologists, social workers, and nurses). Such specification of the basis for the evidence provided will allow for greater understanding of the quality of the evidence as support for a judgment regarding financial capability.

Systematic Identification of Adult SSA Beneficiaries at Risk for Financial Incapability

The following conclusions and recommendations address systematic identification of individuals who are risk for financial incapability.

---

[7] This would include, to the extent possible, the beneficiary's perspective on the relationship as well as the informant's.

Risk Criteria

Reliance on diagnostic criteria alone for determining financial (in)capability is inadequate for a number of reasons, including the likelihood of identifying too many people as incapable in some diagnostic categories and missing people in others, a central concern raised by the OIG-SSA reports. Identification of easy-to-apply, efficient approaches, including the development of screening criteria, that could be incorporated into the disability application process to identify people at high risk for incapability would be valuable in helping to ensure that potentially incapable beneficiaries receive further evaluation.

Recommendation 2. The U.S. Social Security Administration should create a data-driven process to support the development of approaches, including screening criteria, for identifying people at high risk for financial incapability.

SSA has the opportunity, whether through the development of formal screening criteria or other approaches (e.g., identifying risk markers to inform the judgment of field officers), to improve its ability to identify beneficiaries who may lack financial capability. The committee envisions the development of a model based on existing data, such as age, gender, impairment code assigned by SSA, and education level, to identify predictors of incapability. The resulting model could be refined and its reliability and validity improved through pilot projects involving samples of beneficiaries who would undergo more detailed assessments of capability. Prior to large-scale implementation, the success of the resulting approach in identifying incapable beneficiaries who would not otherwise have been found could be tested.

Dual Beneficiaries

A 2012 SSA-OIG report indicated that more than 6,000 individuals who were receiving benefits from both the SSI and SSDI programs had been assigned a representative payee in one program but not the other. In addition, SSA beneficiaries also may receive benefits from another federal agency, such as the VA or OPM. While acknowledging the potential technological, legal, and procedural challenges to data sharing, the committee concludes that sharing information about incapability determinations within SSA and among relevant federal agencies could increase the likelihood of each agency's identifying potentially incapable beneficiaries. Agencies could then use the information to trigger their own capability assessments of beneficiaries identified in this way.

Recommendation 3. The U.S. Social Security Administration (SSA) should ensure intra-agency communication regarding capability determinations within its different programs. In addition, SSA, the U.S. Department of Veterans Affairs, and other relevant federal agencies should assess the extent of inconsistency in the identification of beneficiaries who are incapable among persons receiving benefits from more than one agency. Based on the findings of this assessment, the relevant agencies should explore mechanisms to facilitate ongoing interagency communication regarding the capability of beneficiaries.

OPM, for example, uses computerized matching to identify beneficiaries who receive other federal benefits. Although such matching is used primarily to analyze whether benefits from other programs may affect OPM benefits, a process of this sort can also provide information that indicates whether other programs have identified the beneficiary as having impaired capability.

Responding to Changes in Capability Over Time

Many psychiatric and cognitive conditions are characterized by progression or fluctuation over time in the presence, severity, and nature of symptoms. Such changes suggest the value of a process for periodic reassessment of a beneficiary's capability. SSA's lack of a formal process for periodically reviewing a beneficiary's capability is a significant weakness. Some mechanism for periodic reassessment is needed to ensure that beneficiaries with fluctuating, deteriorating, or improving financial capability are classified accurately. Accordingly, the committee makes the following recommendation:

Recommendation 4. The U.S. Social Security Administration should develop systematic mechanisms for recognizing and responding to changes in beneficiaries' capability over time.

For disability beneficiaries, SSA procedures call for periodic continuing disability reviews (CDRs). Although CDRs provide an opportunity for capability (re)assessments, their purpose is to identify any changes (improvements) in the medical basis for a beneficiary's disability award. Thus, even if the CDRs were to occur on schedule, they would not fully serve the purpose of reassessment of financial capability. SSA could apply the same principle used in the CDR process to develop an analogous process for recognizing and responding to changes in capability over time. Reassessments initially could be targeted toward (1) beneficiaries who had been determined to be incapable but who might improve over time as their conditions or environmental supports changed; and (2) beneficiaries who, although capable, were at risk for becoming incapable as their condition progressed or their environment changed. As screening criteria or other systematic methods for identifying people at high risk for financial incapability were developed, they might be used to broaden the target population for periodic reassessment.

In addition, beneficiaries, family members, representative payees, and professionals who were likely to come into contact with beneficiaries could be alerted systematically to notify SSA if they believed that beneficiaries' capability had changed so as to warrant redetermination. SSA might also implement a process to survey payees and/or beneficiaries periodically, similar to that of OPM, integrating screening questions that could trigger the need to further investigate the beneficiary's financial capability.

Supervised Direct Payment

By their nature, SSA capability determinations are dichotomous; that is, beneficiaries are either capable or incapable of managing or directing the management of their benefits. As noted, however, a beneficiary's capability may change as a result of progressive or temporary diminution or improvement in his or her financial competence and performance over time. When information available about a beneficiary's financial performance is insufficient to determine the need to appoint a representative payee, the use of a supervised direct payment option may be helpful. Under such a model, benefits are paid directly to the beneficiary, but an individual is designated to supervise the beneficiary's expenditures. Reassessment after a trial period during which the beneficiary's use of benefits is observed and assessed permits more accurate determination of the beneficiary's capability in indeterminate or borderline cases.

Supervised direct payment may have other advantages. By adopting a supported decision-making model, supervisors can provide guidance and instruction to beneficiaries on managing their benefits and help respond to the challenges posed by the fluctuations in some beneficiaries' financial competence and performance. Supported decision making encourages beneficiaries' expression of preferences, beliefs, and values; allows collaboration in decision making; and provides opportunities for beneficiaries to make independent decisions whenever possible. Appropriate use of this approach may provide a beneficiary with greater control over his or her life than would be the case for someone without such support. Supervised direct payment may enable some beneficiaries who might otherwise require the appointment of a representative payee to manage or direct the management of their benefits to meet their basic needs, thus maximizing their decisional autonomy. For these reasons, the committee makes the following recommendation:

Recommendation 5. The U.S. Social Security Administration should implement a demonstration project to evaluate the efficacy of a supervised direct payment option for qualified beneficiaries.

"Qualified beneficiaries" refers to two groups of individuals. The first is beneficiaries who may be incapable of managing or directing the management of their benefits but for whom there is insufficient information regarding financial performance to render a determination. The second is beneficiaries who are determined by SSA to be incapable, but who either display financial performance in some but not all areas of benefit management or successfully manage their benefits some but not all of the time. The VA's supervised direct payment option for individuals who are determined to be incompetent but able to manage benefits with supervision provides a model for such an approach. Instead of the VA's appointing a fiduciary for such individuals, they receive their benefits directly but under the supervision of a Veterans Service Center Manager. This approach could provide a model for a demonstration project by SSA.

Program Evaluation

Data are limited on the effectiveness of current SSA processes for identifying beneficiaries who should be evaluated for capability and on the accuracy of capability determinations among those identified for evaluation. Reports issued by OIG-SSA in 2004, 2010, and 2012 suggest that SSA's current capability determination process fails to identify all the beneficiaries who would benefit from the appointment of a representative payee. The committee has made a number of recommendations that could increase the identification of beneficiaries in need of a representative payee. Without baseline data and ongoing data collection, however, the effectiveness of current policies or the impact of the recommended changes cannot be evaluated. The committee therefore makes the following recommendation:

Recommendation 6. The U.S. Social Security Administration should develop and implement an ongoing measurement and evaluation process to quantify and track the accuracy of capability determinations and to inform and improve its policies and procedures for identifying beneficiaries who are incapable of managing or directing the management of their benefits.

The measurement and evaluation process envisioned in the present report would need to be designed and carried out by trained experts (whether in house or external) with detailed knowledge of SSA work flow and procedures. Such a process could comprise a variety of steps, including assessments of the interrater reliability of the capability determination process, in-depth assessments of selected beneficiaries to determine the accuracy of earlier determinations, and evaluations of the impact of the recommendations in this report (e.g., guidance on the evidence to be provided for capability determinations). A robust measurement and evaluation process would provide substantial and much-needed insight into what SSA is currently doing well and what it may, at reasonable cost, be able to do significantly better.

1

Introduction

The U.S. Social Security Administration (SSA) administers the Old-Age, Survivors, and Disability Insurance (OASDI) and Supplemental Security Income (SSI) programs, providing benefits to approximately 64 million Americans (SSA, 2015d). Within OASDI, Old-Age and Survivors Insurance (OASI) pays benefits to retired workers who have paid into the program and their dependents and survivors, while Social Security Disability Insurance (SSDI) provides benefits to adults with disabilities who have worked and paid into the Disability Insurance trust fund and to their spouses and adult children who are unable to work because of disability.[1] SSI, a means-tested program based on income and financial assets, provides income assistance from U.S. Treasury general funds to adults aged 65 or older, individuals who are blind, and disabled adults and children (SSA, 2015a). As of December 2014, approximately 48 million individuals received OASI benefits, about 11 million received SSDI benefits, and about 8 million received assistance through the SSI program. Of the roughly 64 million beneficiaries, approximately 3 million received benefits through both OASDI and SSI (SSA, 2015d).

The Social Security Act Amendments of 1939 gave the Commissioner of Social Security the authority to make benefit payments to an individual

[1] Disabled beneficiaries who are now adults but became disabled prior to age 22, which SSA refers to as *disabled adult child beneficiaries*, receive benefits based on their parents' Social Security earnings record. To be eligible for disabled widow(er) benefits, the widow(er) must be between the ages of 50 and 59, prove his or her relationship to the disabled worker, and demonstrate his or her disability.

or organization other than the beneficiary when doing so would serve the beneficiary's interests. This so-called *representative payee* must use the benefits in the beneficiary's interest, although he or she may directly distribute small portions of the payment to the beneficiary.[2] To determine the need for a representative payee, SSA must make a *capability determination*, that is, a determination as to whether the beneficiary is capable of managing or directing the management of his or her benefits. When there is some indication that a beneficiary may not be able to manage or direct the management of his or her benefits, evidence of capability/incapability must be developed (i.e., gathered and evaluated). SSA designates three categories of evidence in the capability determination process: legal, medical, and lay.[3]

Legal evidence comprises findings regarding competence by the courts. SSA beneficiaries who have been declared legally incompetent through a court order are required to receive their funds through a representative payee. When no such court order exists, medical and lay evidence are developed. Medical evidence comprises information about a person's physical or mental condition (e.g., medical signs and laboratory findings, medical history and treatment records, opinions from medical sources) that sheds light on a beneficiary's ability to manage or direct the management of funds, based on an examination of the beneficiary by a physician, psychologist, or other qualified medical practitioner. Lay evidence comprises anything other than legal or medical evidence that provides material and relevant facts as to the beneficiary's ability to manage or direct the management of funds to meet his or her basic needs. Such evidence can be provided by anyone with direct knowledge of facts or circumstances regarding the beneficiary in his or her daily life; this may include nonprofessionals (e.g., relatives, friends, neighbors) and health care and social service professionals (e.g., social workers, occupational therapists, rehabilitation specialists, adult protective services workers). All relevant evidence is evaluated, and a determination is made as to whether the beneficiary is capable. Upon determination that a beneficiary is incapable, SSA informs the beneficiary that it has determined he or she needs a representative payee, provides the name of the proposed representative payee, and apprises the beneficiary of his or her appeal rights (SSA's process for capability determinations is discussed in greater detail in Chapter 2).

SSA asked the Institute of Medicine of the National Academies of Sciences, Engineering, and Medicine (the Academies) to convene a committee of experts with relevant expertise to evaluate SSA's capability determination

[2] This sentence has been modified from the prepublication version of the report.

[3] To ensure consistency with SSA's language and allow for comparisons between SSA's capability determination process and that of other agencies and organizations, the committee discusses evidence of capability in accordance with this terminology.

process for adult beneficiaries and provide recommendations for improving the accuracy and efficiency of the agency's policy and procedures for making these determinations (see Box 1-1 for the committee's full statement of task). In carrying out this task, the committee was asked to address several specific topics, including capability determination processes used in similar benefit programs, requisite abilities for managing or directing the management of benefits, methods and measures for assessing capability, the use of capacity assessment tools, appropriate roles for SSA and state Disability Determination Services employees, and effects on the beneficiary of appointing a representative payee. The 12-member committee included experts in the areas of psychology, neuropsychology, psychiatry, social work, occupational therapy and rehabilitation, behavioral economics, bioethics, and law (see Appendix D for biographical sketches of the committee members). This report presents the results of the committee's efforts, including its findings, conclusions, and recommendations.

BOX 1-1
Statement of Task

An ad hoc committee will conduct a study to evaluate the U.S. Social Security Administration's (SSA's) capability determination process for adult beneficiaries. In carrying out this task, the committee will

1. Familiarize itself with SSA's current policy and procedures for capability determinations for adult beneficiaries;
2. Provide an overview of the capability determination processes in at least three similar benefit programs (at least one government program and one private-sector program);
3. Compare SSA's program to these other programs; and
4. Provide recommendations to improve the accuracy and efficiency of SSA's policy and procedures for capability determinations.

To accomplish these objectives, the committee shall consider the following topics:

1. Capability determination processes used by other similar benefit programs;
2. Abilities required to manage, and direct the management of, benefits;
3. Effective methods and measures for assessing capability;
4. Use of capacity assessments tools;
5. Appropriate roles of SSA employees, state Disability Determination Services employees, and others in making capability determinations; and
6. Effects of SSA's decision to appoint a payee on the beneficiary.

CONTEXT

Prior to 1956, SSA was responsible primarily for providing benefits to eligible retirees and their families. Among retired adult beneficiaries, 1.4 percent (527,635 of 39 million) had a representative payee as of December 2014 (SSA, 2015a). However, subsequent expansions of the Social Security program to include disability benefits (1956) and SSI payments (1974) not only increased the number of beneficiaries but also significantly altered the demographics of those receiving benefits. The inclusion of persons with disabilities, those who are blind, and adults aged 65 or older with limited income and resources among those receiving benefits increased the number of beneficiaries in need of a representative payee. In December 2014, more than 3.5 million adults received SSDI benefits (1.7 million[4]) or SSI payments (1.8 million) through a representative payee, nearly seven times the number of retired adult beneficiaries with representative payees. (See Tables 1-1 and 1-2 for the number of beneficiaries with a representative payee by type of beneficiary.) Approximately 160,000 new representative payees are appointed each year (Stanton, 2015).

Recent audits by SSA's Office of the Inspector General (OIG-SSA) found beneficiaries with mental impairments (SSA OIG, 2012) and beneficiaries of advanced age (over age 85) (SSA OIG, 2010) who were in need of a representative payee but were not identified as such. Comments presented to the committee in open session suggest that SSA's capability determinations are more likely to miss beneficiaries who need a representative payee than to require a representative payee unnecessarily (Beard, 2015; Payne, 2015; Stanton, 2015). Based on demographic changes in the population of SSA beneficiaries, especially growth in the retired-worker population and the increasing percentage of beneficiaries aged 85 and older, Anguelov and colleagues (2015) project that the number of adult OASDI beneficiaries and SSI recipients in need of a representative payee will increase by 620,000 (21.1 percent) by 2035.[5]

The primary goal of representative payment is to ensure that benefits are expended in the best interests of the beneficiary.[6] Recognizing the

[4] This number includes disabled adult beneficiaries, disabled widow(er) beneficiaries, and disabled adult child beneficiaries.

[5] Based on the 2013 population of beneficiaries aged 18 or older who were not receiving benefits as disabled adult children or as students aged 18-19.

[6] The committee recognizes the subjective nature of determining whether individuals' choices serve their "best interests" with regard to financial decisions. Given the focus of this report (i.e., determination of capability to manage SSA benefits), the committee adopted the standard for serving one's best interests of satisfying the basic needs of food, shelter, and clothing. This standard is consistent with SSA's guidance to employees and representative payees (SSA, 2012, 2015e, n.d.-a,b), and is intended to be minimally restrictive of the liberty of beneficiaries to manage their own affairs.

TABLE 1-1 Characteristics of Old-Age, Survivors, and Disability Insurance Beneficiaries with Representative Payees, December 2014

		Beneficiaries with Representative Payees	
Type of Beneficiary	All Beneficiaries	Number	Percentage
Adults	54,651,944	1,627,244	3.0
Retired	39,008,771	527,635	1.4
Spouses	2,452,435	22,999	0.9
Nondisabled widow(er)s	3,978,349	115,821	2.9
Disabled	8,954,518	946,015	10.6
Disabled widow(er)s	257,871	14,774	5.7
Children	4,355,214	3,944,251	90.6
Under 18	3,166,362	3,164,001	99.9
Disabled adult children	1,048,879	774,621	73.9
Students, aged 18-19	139,973	5,629	4.0
Total	59,007,158	5,571,495	9.4

SOURCE: SSA, 2015a, Table 5.L1.

TABLE 1-2 Number and Percentage Distribution of Supplemental Security Income (SSI) Recipients with Representative Payees Receiving Federally Administered Payments, by Eligibility Category and Age, December 2014

		Beneficiaries with Representative Payees	
Category and Age	All Beneficiaries	Number	Percentage
Category			
Aged	1,151,940	53,463	4.6
Blind	67,383	19,839	29.4
Disabled	7,116,381	3,080,664	43.3
Age			
Under 18	1,299,761	1,298,826	99.9
18-64	4,913,072	1,658,536	33.8
65 or older*	2,122,871	196,604	9.3
Total	8,335,704	3,153,966	37.8

* Includes blind persons and disabled persons aged 65 or older.
SOURCE: SSA, 2015a, Table 7.E4.

importance of the representative payee program to the well-being of beneficiaries in need, SSA often has sought to improve various aspects of the program, conducting internal reviews and seeking expert advice from external sources. In 1995, SSA chartered the Representative Payment Advisory Committee (1996) to review the full spectrum of SSA's representative payment program and "provide input into designing a better program" (p. vii). In 2004, SSA charged the Academies with examining issues related to potential misuse of payments to representative payees, with the final report of that study issued in 2007 (NRC, 2007). OIG-SSA has conducted multiple audits of the representative payee program with respect to potential misuse of benefits (SSA OIG, 2008) and SSA's process for determining whether a beneficiary is capable of managing his or her benefits (SSA OIG, 2004, 2010, 2012).

CLARIFICATION OF STUDY SCOPE

The committee was tasked with evaluating SSA's capability determination process for adult beneficiaries. As evidenced in Tables 1-1 and 1-2, SSA serves a diverse population, including adults with disabilities; disabled adult children; and nondisabled adults, including aged SSI recipients and retirement beneficiaries. Table 1-3 presents the number and percentage of adult beneficiaries in these three groups with representative payees.

At the committee's first meeting, SSA representatives clarified that the committee should focus on adults with disabilities (Stanton, 2015).[7] This group may include disabled adult children; however, an examination of the dynamics unique to the transitional process from child to adult beneficiary is beyond the scope of this study (Stanton, 2015). SSA acknowledged that adults receiving retirement benefits may be determined incapable and have a representative payee appointed. Where applicable, therefore, results of the present study also may provide guidance on capability determinations for these individuals. However, issues unique to retirement beneficiaries were not considered to be within the scope of this study (Stanton, 2015). For example, identifying retirement beneficiaries who may need a representative payee presents a significant challenge because in contrast with disability applicants, SSA rarely has contact with these individuals, and therefore may be unlikely to become aware of those who may require a representative payee. Indeed, OIG-SSA estimated that approximately 1 million beneficiaries over the age of 85 were receiving direct payment but were incapable of managing their benefits (SSA OIG, 2010).

[7] The parameters stated herein were confirmed by Joanna Firman, SSA's contracting officer's technical representative, at the committee's first meeting.

TABLE 1-3 Number and Percentage of Adult Beneficiaries with Representative Payees by Type, December 2014

		Beneficiaries with Representative Payees	
Type of Beneficiary	All Beneficiaries	Number	Percentage
Adults with disabilities	15,096,392	2,762,456	18.3
OASDI	9,212,389	960,789	10.4
SSI (blindness or disability)	5,884,003	1,801,667	30.6
Disabled adult children	1,048,879	774,621	73.9
Nondisabled adults	46,591,495	618,871	1.3
OASDI	45,439,555	565,408	1.2
SSI (aged)	1,151,940	53,463	4.6

SOURCE: SSA, 2015a (calculated from Tables 5.L1 and 7.E4).

TERMINOLOGY AND CONCEPTUAL MODEL

The terms *ability*, *capability*, *capacity*, and *competency* often are used interchangeably, and their interpretation may vary across disciplines, with nuances that may be difficult to distinguish for the lay reader. At its second meeting, for example, the committee heard from a number of experts who referred to similar concepts using each of these terms. *Financial capacity* (Marson, 2015), *decision-making capacity* (Karlawish, 2015), and *the capability to manage SSI and SSDI benefits* (Rosen, 2015) were discussed, as was the U.S. Department of Veterans Affairs (VA) process for incompetency determinations (Flohr and Lewis, 2015).

Early in the study process, the committee identified the need to distinguish among these and other commonly used terms and to define each in the context of this study to ensure clarity and consistency in its deliberations and throughout this report. Terminology that is fundamental to the committee's report is described herein. Appendix B contains a glossary of definitions for a number of terms that are particularly relevant to the committee's work. In its guidelines, SSA (2015b) defines *capability* as

> a beneficiary's ability to manage or direct the management of his [or] her Social Security funds. . . . A beneficiary who exercises direct involvement, control and choice in identifying, accessing and managing services to meet his/her personal and other needs is capable and must be paid directly.

Managing one's own funds means one is fully and independently responsible for disbursing the funds in a way that routinely[8] meets one's basic needs. Even if someone is not capable of fully and independently managing his or her own funds, however, that person may still be capable of *directing the management* of the funds by someone else. SSA also refers to this as *self-direction*, "a service delivery system whereby families, elderly beneficiaries, or beneficiaries with disabilities have high levels of direct involvement, control and choice in identifying, accessing and managing the services they obtain to meet their personal assistance and other health related needs" (SSA, 2015c). For example, individuals with mental impairments may be able to direct others to manage their funds based on their goals, such as paying rent on time so as not to lose their apartment, even though they are not able to perform the day-to-day tasks necessary to achieve those goals. Similarly, individuals who are mentally capable of managing their own funds but have a physical impairment, such as quadriplegia or an inability to speak, that makes them physically unable to accomplish the tasks required to do so may still be able to direct someone else to perform those tasks.

In the context of SSA capability determinations, the question is really one of *financial capability*—managing or directing the management of one's funds in a way that routinely meets one's best interests. For SSA, the determination of capability is a dichotomous decision, akin to the legal definition of incompetence[9]: one either is or is not capable. Thus, *incapability* is a determination that an individual beneficiary is unable to manage or direct the management of his or her benefits as a result of mental impairment or, sometimes, physical disability. Throughout this report, discussions of financial capability refer specifically to the dichotomous decision regarding whether a beneficiary is able to manage or direct the management of his or her benefits. The process for making this determination relies on evaluation of the beneficiary's *financial performance* and/or *financial competence* (see Figure 1-1).

Financial Competence and Financial Performance

A fundamental distinction articulated first in linguistic theory but with broader application differentiates between "*competence* (the speaker-hearer's knowledge of his language) and *performance* (the actual use of

[8] The committee recognizes that circumstances and personal preferences at times may require or lead someone to forgo a basic need, such as food. Nevertheless, the individual's overall behavior may still meet his or her basic needs.

[9] In legal terms, *incompetency* refers to a determination by the courts that an individual is unable to manage his or her affairs as a result of mental impairment or sometimes physical disability. SSA uses the term *legally incompetent* to refer to one subset of beneficiaries who will automatically receive a representative payee.

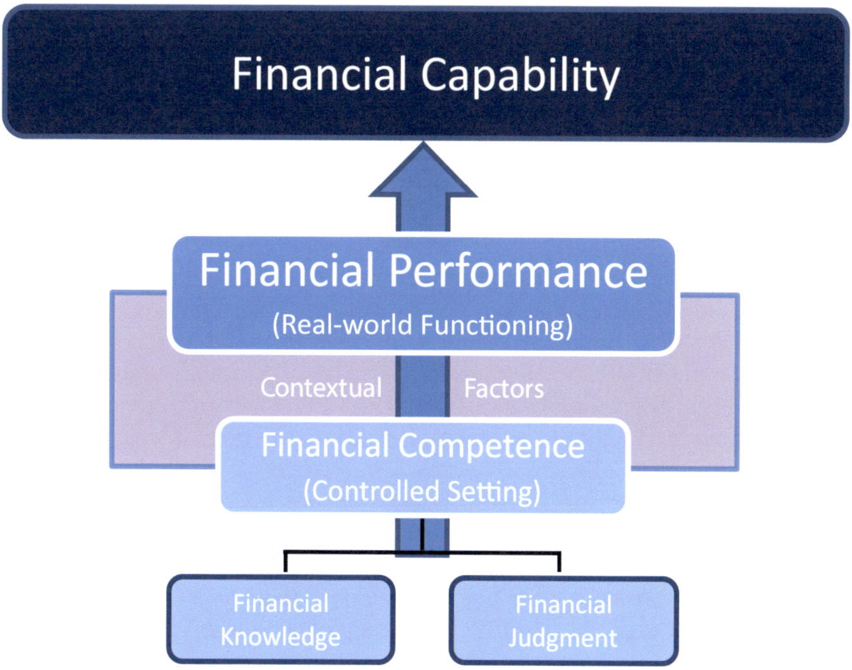

FIGURE 1-1 Conceptual model of financial capability.

language in concrete situations)" (Chomsky, 1965, p. 4). Similarly, the committee defines *financial performance* as an individual's degree of success in handling financial demands in the context of the stresses, supports, contextual cues, and resources in his or her actual environment. *Financial competence* refers to financial skills one possesses, as demonstrated through *financial knowledge* and *financial judgment*, typically assessed in a controlled (e.g., office or other clinical) setting.

Financial knowledge is possession of the declarative knowledge (i.e., information that a person knows) and procedural knowledge (i.e., knowing how to perform a task) required to manage one's finances. Examples of such declarative and procedural knowledge include the concept of money, values of currency, making change, check writing, use of ATMs (automated teller machines), and online banking procedures. *Financial judgment* is possession of the abilities (understanding, reasoning, and appreciation) needed to make financial decisions and choices that serve the individual's best interests.

A high degree of financial performance requires not only sufficient levels of *financial competence*, but also possession of the abilities required to implement financial decisions in everyday life (e.g., impulse control, anxiety management, and resistance to external pressures) and the opportunity to exercise those abilities in the real world.

Effects of Context on Competence and Performance

The World Health Organization's (WHO's) *International Classification of Functioning, Disability and Health* conceives of functioning and disability "as a dynamic interaction between health conditions (diseases, disorders, injuries, traumas, etc.) and contextual factors" (WHO, 2001, p. 8). Underlying financial competence and financial performance, as depicted in the committee's conceptual model of financial capability (see Figure 1-1), is the individual's *context*, the personal and environmental factors that may facilitate or hinder functioning, either independently or in their interaction. Personal factors are features of an individual that may affect his or her functioning, such as gender, age, social background, education, past and current experience, and the like (WHO, 2001, p. 17). Environmental factors are "features of the physical, social, and attitudinal environment in which people live and conduct their lives" (WHO, 2001, p. 16), such as acute or chronic stressors, social supports, financial and emotional resources, opportunities, and barriers.

The influence of such factors on a beneficiary may result in performance that is better or worse than expected based on the person's level of financial competence. Therefore, financial competence can be viewed as the potential for, but not necessarily determinative of, adequate (i.e., satisfactory and sufficient to fulfill a specified requirement or purpose) financial performance. An individual may be financially competent (i.e., possess and demonstrate financial knowledge and judgment) in an office or clinical setting but be unable to exercise his or her financial knowledge, skills, and judgment in a real-world setting. Conversely, a person may fail to demonstrate financial knowledge or judgment in a controlled setting but be able to perform capably with the assistance of support systems in his or her environment. The effects of context on financial competence and performance are discussed in greater detail in Chapter 3.

Box 1-2 provides the working definitions for key terms used by the committee in its deliberations and throughout this report.

A Note on Financial Literacy

It is worth briefly noting an evolving distinction in the literature between *financial capability* and *financial literacy*, although the terms also are often used synonymously (Sherraden, 2013). Generally, financial capability is a broader notion that encompasses financial literacy. Whereas

BOX 1-2
Key Terms Defined

Context: personal factors (e.g., gender, age, social background, education, past and current experience) and environmental factors (acute or chronic stressors, social supports, financial and emotional resources, opportunities, and barriers) that may facilitate or hinder functioning

Financial capability: the management or direction of the management of one's funds in a way that routinely meets one's best interests

Financial competence: the financial skills one possesses, as demonstrated through financial knowledge and financial judgment, typically assessed in a controlled (e.g., office or clinical) setting

Financial judgment: possession of the abilities (understanding, reasoning, and appreciation) needed to make financial decisions and choices that serve the individual's best interests

Financial knowledge: possession of the declarative and procedural knowledge required to manage one's finances

Financial performance: the degree of success in handling financial demands in the context of the stresses, supports, contextual cues, and resources in the individual's actual environment

Lay evidence: any evidence other than legal or medical evidence that provides material and relevant facts as to the beneficiary's ability to manage or direct the management of funds and meet his or her basic needs

Legal evidence: findings by the courts regarding competence

Medical evidence: information about a person's physical or mental condition (e.g., medical signs and laboratory findings, medical history and treatment records, opinions from medical sources) that sheds light on a beneficiary's ability to manage or direct the management of funds, based on an examination of the beneficiary by a physician, psychologist, or other qualified medical practitioner

financial literacy "typically refers to the knowledge and skills needed to make sound financial decisions," financial capability also includes "access to financial services, behavioral factors, social influences, and emotions" (Collins, 2013, p. 1). Moving from financial literacy to financial capability entails moving from an individual's possession of financial knowledge and skills (capacity) to his or her financial functioning in the real world (performance). The inclusion of financial judgment and financial performance (in addition to financial knowledge) in the committee's concept of financial capability is consistent with this distinction between financial literacy and financial capability. In the committee's model, financial literacy would be most akin to financial knowledge, the term the committee uses in discussing the underlying declarative and procedural knowledge required to manage one's finances.

STUDY APPROACH

The committee conducted an extensive review of the literature pertaining to financial capability. This review began with an English-, German-, Spanish-, and Hebrew-language[10] search of online databases, including PubMed, Embase, Medline, Health and Psychological Instruments, Scopus, Web of Science, and ProQuest. Committee members and project staff identified additional literature and other resources using traditional academic research methods and online searches throughout the course of the study.

The committee used a variety of sources to supplement its review of the literature. It met in person five times, and held two public workshops and two public teleconferences to hear from invited experts in areas pertinent to the study. Speakers at the workshops included experts on financial capability assessment; the SSA representative payee system, its process, and its impacts on the beneficiary; abilities required to manage or direct the management of benefits; and the effects of everyday surroundings on financial performance. The committee also heard from representatives of SSA, state Disability Determination Services, and the National Association of Disability Examiners about the SSA capability determination process and procedures for adult beneficiaries with disabilities, as well as representatives from the VA, the U.S. Office of Personnel Management (OPM), and the Canada Pension Plan (CPP) and the Old Age Security program regarding similar processes of each of these organizations. Finally, with America's Health Insurance Plans (AHIP)[11] acting as an intermediary, the committee received information compiled from five disability income protection insurers regarding their approaches to determining capability.

REPORT ORGANIZATION

In the following chapters, the committee provides a description of SSA's current policy and processes for capability determinations, along with the policies and processes of similar programs in other government agencies and nongovernmental organizations, including the VA, OPM, CPP and the Old Age Security program, and the private insurance industry (Chapter 2); effects of the appointment of representative payees on beneficiaries (Chapter 3); a conceptual overview of the components of financial capability and the underlying cognitive and behavioral processes (Chapter 4); and an examination of methods and measures for assessing financial capability, including formal assessment instruments designed for this purpose and the individuals best suited to performing the assessment

[10] Languages in which committee members were fluent.

[11] AHIP is the national trade association representing the health insurance industry.

(Chapter 5). Within each chapter, the committee provides findings and conclusions relevant to the respective topics. In Chapter 6, the committee presents its overall conclusions and recommendations, which it hopes will assist SSA in its ongoing endeavor to improve its benefit programs and better serve those who rely on them.

REFERENCES

Anguelov, C. E., G. Ravida, and R. R. Weathers II. 2015. Adult OASDI beneficiaries and SSI recipients who need representative payees: Projections for 2025 and 2035. *Social Security Bulletin* 75(2). https://www.ssa.gov/policy/docs/ssb/v75n2/v75n2p1.html (accessed February 22, 2016).

Beard, A. 2015. Description of the capability determination process and the field office role in the process. Presentation to the Committee to Evaluate the Social Security Administration's Capability Determination Process for Adult Beneficiaries, February 3, Washington, DC.

Chomsky, N. 1965. *Aspects of the theory of syntax*. Cambridge, MA: MIT Press.

Collins, J. M. 2013. Analyzing the financial capability of people in Wisconsin. *Issue Briefs: Family Financial Education 2013-04*. http://fyi.uwex.edu/financialseries/files/2013/04/April_2013_Fin_Cap1.pdf (accessed September 11, 2015).

Flohr, B., and C. Lewis. 2015. Veterans Benefits Administration incompetency determinations. Presentation to the Committee to Evaluate the Social Security Administration's Capability Determination Process for Adult Beneficiaries, April 21, Washington, DC.

Karlawish, J. 2015. Measuring everyday decision-making capacity. Presentation to the Committee to Evaluate the Social Security Administration's Capability Determination Process for Adult Beneficiaries, April 21, Washington, DC.

Marson, D. C. 2015. Assessing financial capacity: A brief overview. Presentation to the Committee to Evaluate the Social Security Administration's Capability Determination Process for Adult Beneficiaries, April 21, Washington, DC.

NRC (National Research Council). 2007. *Improving the Social Security representative payee program: Serving beneficiaries and minimizing misuse*. Washington, DC: The National Academies Press.

Payne, D. 2015. Description of the disability determination services' role in the capability determination process. Presentation to the Committee to Evaluate the Social Security Administration's Capability Determination Process for Adult Beneficiaries, February 3, Washington, DC.

Representative Payment Advisory Committee. 1996. *Final report of the Representative Payment Advisory Committee*.

Rosen, M. I. 2015. Data-driven approaches to assessing which SSI/SSDI recipients are capable of managing their benefits. Presentation to the Committee to Evaluate the Social Security Administration's Capability Determination Process for Adult Beneficiaries, April 21, Washington, DC.

Sherraden, M. S. 2013. Building blocks of financial capability. In *Financial education and capability: Research, education, policy, and practice*, edited by J. Birkenmaier, M. Sherraden, and J. Curley. New York: Oxford University Press. Pp. 3-43.

SSA (U.S. Social Security Administration). 2012. *GN 00602.001 Use of benefits*. https://secure.ssa.gov/apps10/poms.nsf/lnx/0200602001 (accessed January 29, 2016).

SSA. 2015a. *Annual statistical supplement*. https://www.socialsecurity.gov/policy/docs/statcomps/supplement/2015/index.html (accessed February 8, 2016).

SSA. 2015b. *GN 00502.010 Capability determination—overview*. https://secure.ssa.gov/poms.nsf/lnx/0200502010 (accessed August 4, 2015).

SSA. 2015c. *GN 00502.020 Determining capability—adult beneficiaries*. https://secure.ssa.gov/poms.nsf/lnx/0200502020 (accessed December 15, 2015).

SSA. 2015d. *Fast facts and figures about Social Security, 2015*. https://www.socialsecurity.gov/policy/docs/chartbooks/fast_facts/2015/fast_facts15.pdf (accessed January 24, 2016).

SSA. 2015e. *Understanding Supplemental Security Income Representative Payee Program—2015 edition*. https://www.socialsecurity.gov/ssi/text-repayee-ussi.htm (accessed January 29, 2016).

SSA. n.d.-a. *Frequently asked questions (FAQs) for representative payees*. https://www.ssa.gov/payee/faqrep.htm#&a0=9 (accessed January 29, 2016).

SSA. n.d.-b. *Social Security: A guide for representative payees*. https://www.ssa.gov/pubs/EN-05-10076.pdf (accessed October 30, 2015).

SSA OIG (Office of the Inspector General). 2004. *The Social Security Administration's representative payee selection process*. http://oig.ssa.gov/sites/default/files/audit/full/pdf/A-01-04-14008.pdf (accessed January 29, 2016).

SSA OIG. 2008. *Beneficiary and recipient use of "in care of" addresses*. http://oig.ssa.gov/sites/default/files/audit/full/pdf/A-06-08-18015_0.pdf (accessed January 29, 2016).

SSA OIG. 2010. *Aged beneficiaries in need of representative payees*. http://oig.ssa.gov/sites/default/files/audit/full/pdf/A-09-09-29002.pdf (accessed January 29, 2016).

SSA OIG. 2012. *Disabled individuals with mental impairments in need of a representative payee*. http://oig.ssa.gov/sites/default/files/audit/full/pdf/A-07-11-11110.pdf (accessed January 29, 2016).

Stanton, S. 2015. Opening remarks and overview of the SSA capability determination process. Presentation to the Committee to Evaluate the Social Security Administration's Capability Determination Process for Adult Beneficiaries, February 3, Washington, DC.

WHO (World Health Organization). 2001. *International Classification of Functioning, Disability and Health (ICF)*. Geneva, Switzerland: WHO.

2

Review of the Social Security Administration and Other Selected Capability Determination Processes

As part of its statement of task, the committee was asked to "familiarize itself with the U.S. Social Security Administration's (SSA's) current policy and procedures for capability determinations for adult beneficiaries; provide an overview of the capability determination processes in at least three similar programs (at least one government and one private sector program); [and] compare SSA's program to these other programs." To meet these objectives, the committee examined current policies and procedures of and spoke with representatives from SSA, the U.S. Department of Veterans Affairs (VA), the U.S. Office of Personnel Management (OPM), and Service Canada.[1] Additionally, with America's Health Insurance Plans (AHIP) serving as an intermediary, the committee was provided with information compiled from five disability income protection insurers.

Some SSA beneficiaries also receive benefits from the VA or OPM. Because each of these agencies has its own policies and procedures for determining whether beneficiaries are capable of managing their benefits, they may reach different conclusions about an individual's capability. Flohr and Lewis (2015) report that there is no formal method for the exchange of information between SSA and the VA with regard to beneficiaries found incompetent. However, they also note that in certain cases, the VA field examiners recommend that the VA-appointed fiduciary apply to serve in a similar role for SSA benefits. The OPM program uses computerized matching with

[1] A representative of the U.S. Railroad Retirement Board was scheduled to present at the committee's first workshop. However, the representative canceled prior to the meeting, and despite the committee's efforts, no further contact was established.

other benefit-paying organizations, including SSA and the U.S. Department of Labor. Although such matching is primarily for analysis of benefit disbursement from other programs that may affect OPM benefits, it may also provide information that brings capability into question (Spear, 2015).

The current chapter explores and compares these organizations' processes and policies for determining capability.[2] Annex Table 2-1 at the end of this chapter summarizes information about each of these programs and allows cross-program comparisons.

OVERVIEW OF SSA AND OTHER SELECTED PROGRAMS

The Social Security Act grants the commissioner of Social Security authority to make benefit payments to an individual or organization other than the beneficiary, a so-called representative payee, when it would serve the beneficiary's best interests. Such an arrangement is made for beneficiaries whom SSA has deemed incapable of managing or directing the management of their benefits and in need of assistance to ensure that their basic needs (i.e., shelter, food, and clothing) are being met.

As of December 2014, approximately 54.65 million adults were receiving Old-Age, Survivors, and Disability Insurance (OASDI) benefits, 1.63 million (3.0 percent) of whom were receiving benefits through a representative payee (SSA, 2015a, Table 5.L1). SSA also administered Supplemental Security Income (SSI) benefits to approximately 7.04 million adults, 1.86 million of whom (26.4 percent) had a representative payee (SSA, 2015a, Table 7.E4). More than 2.55 million adults received benefits from both OASDI and SSI (SSA, 2015d). Of these populations, the great majority of beneficiaries with a representative payee, and the focus of the current report, were adults with disabilities. Table 2-1 shows the number and percentage of adults receiving Social Security Disability Insurance (SSDI) and/or SSI benefits through a representative payee.

The VA is responsible for providing health care and benefits to service members, veterans, and their dependents and survivors. Among these benefits are disability compensation, disability pensions, and service-connected and non-service-connected survivors benefits, all administered by the Veterans Benefits Administration (VBA). As with Social Security, authority is granted to the secretary of the VA to make benefit payments to an individual other than a beneficiary who is found incompetent when doing so

[2] It is important to note that the amount of information provided to or obtained by the committee varied greatly among the programs examined, as reflected in this chapter. Of these programs, SSA and the VA had much information publicly available, while much less information was available on the OPM and Service Canada programs. No information regarding private insurance company programs was publicly available; information provided in this report relies exclusively on the limited information compiled by AHIP.

TABLE 2-1 Number and Percentage of Adult Social Security Disability Insurance (SSDI), Disabled Adult Children SSDI, and Supplemental Security Income (SSI) (Blind or Disabled) Recipients with Representative Payees, December 2014

		Beneficiaries with Representative Payees	
Type of Beneficiary	All Beneficiaries	Number	Percentage
SSDI: Adult	9,212,389	960,789	10.4
Disabled	8,954,518	946,015	10.6
Disabled widow(er)s	257,871	14,774	5.7
SSDI: Disabled adult children	1,048,879	774,621	73.9
SSI: Adult (blindness or disability)*	5,884,003	1,801,667	30.6

NOTE: SSDI = Social Security Disability Insurance; SSI = Supplemental Security Income.
* Numbers calculated from SSA, 2015a, Table 7.E4.
SOURCE: SSA, 2015a, Tables 5.L1 and 7.E4.

appears to be in the beneficiary's best interests.[3] As of September 2014, approximately 3.95 million veterans were receiving disability compensation, and another 300,000 were receiving disability pensions; as of September 2015, approximately 183,000 of these beneficiaries were rated incompetent (Flohr and Lewis, 2015). Table 2-2 shows those conditions with the highest numbers of incompetency ratings.

OPM is responsible for administering and delivering an array of federally authorized benefits and services to its workforce and annuitants. Among these benefits are annuities paid to retirees and their families, administered through the Retirement Services Division, for federal employees eligible for early, voluntary, deferred, or disability retirement. Retirement benefits are paid to approximately 2.5 million annuitants and survivor annuitants each year (Spear, 2015). Federal law permits OPM to make benefit payments to a third party for a beneficiary deemed mentally incompetent or with some other legal disability.[4] Such payment is to be used for the benefit of the annuitant (OPM, n.d.). Currently, there are approximately 16,000 OPM annuitants with representative payees (Spear, 2015).

Employment and Social Development Canada is the Canadian government department responsible for developing, managing, and delivering social programs and services. Among these programs are the Canada Pension Plan (CPP) and Old Age Security (OAS) programs, administered through

[3] 38 USC § 5502.
[4] 5 USC § 8345.

TABLE 2-2 Conditions with Highest Numbers of Incompetency Ratings Within the U.S. Department of Veterans Affairs

Condition	Number
Posttraumatic stress disorder	>15,000
Dementia of unknown etiology	11,000
Schizophrenia, paranoid type	>10,000
Schizophrenia, undifferentiated type	5,700
Dementia, Alzheimer's type	5,400
Major depressive disorder	3,900
Bipolar disorder	2,800
Dementia due to head trauma	2,400
Organic mental disorders	1,200

SOURCE: Flohr and Lewis, 2015.

Service Canada. CPP is a social insurance program based on contributions from workers in Canada that provides pensions and benefits when contributors retire, become disabled, or die. OAS provides benefits to most Canadian citizens or legal residents 65 years of age or older who have lived in Canada for at least 10 years after turning 18, regardless of employment history. In addition to the primary pension, OAS provides the Guaranteed Income Supplement to low-income OAS recipients who live in Canada. Canadian legislation permits the appointment of a person or agency other than the beneficiary, a so-called trustee, to apply for, receive, and administer benefits on behalf of a person who "by reason of infirmity, illness, insanity or other cause, is incapable of managing [his or her] own affairs" (C.R.C., c. 385; R.S.C., 1985, c. O-9). A trustee will be appointed only when doing so is deemed to be in the best interest of the beneficiary, and "no enduring POA [power of attorney] exists or other federally or provincially appointed administration has been put into place" (Service Canada, 2015b).[5] Information on the number of beneficiaries with trustees was unavailable.

As part of its statement of task, the committee was also asked to provide an overview of at least one private-sector program. The committee contacted multiple private insurance companies, but received few responses and no actionable information. However, with assistance from AHIP, which

[5] Service Canada specifically distinguishes an *enduring power of attorney* as a document that "has an explicit provision which states that it will continue or endure despite insanity or incapability of the grantor" (Service Canada, 2015b). A power of attorney without such a provision would not preclude the appointment of a trustee.

conducted outreach to its member companies, the committee received a summary of information compiled from five disability income protection insurers regarding their approaches to determining capability. Respondents reported an overall rate of incapability among claimant populations of less than 5 percent; no respondents offered information regarding rates of incapability determinations by specific diagnosis. Other relevant information provided to the committee by AHIP is discussed throughout this chapter.[6] It is important to note that this information is limited and does not reflect a comprehensive discussion of the various issues involved in the capability determination processes of disability income protection insurers.

DEFINING THE BENEFICIARY'S ABILITY TO MANAGE FUNDS

As noted in Chapter 1, SSA (2003) defines *capability* as "a beneficiary's ability to manage or direct the management of his [or] her Social Security funds." This definition encompasses not only beneficiaries who can directly manage their funds but also those who can participate in the management of their funds by directing others. This second instance is what SSA refers to as *self-direction*, "a service delivery system whereby families, elderly beneficiaries, or beneficiaries with disabilities have high levels of direct involvement, control and choice in identifying, accessing and managing the services they obtain to meet their personal assistance and other health related needs" (SSA, 2015e). If a beneficiary can either manage his or her benefits or direct others in doing so, he or she is deemed capable and must be paid directly. Adult beneficiaries, with the exception of those judged legally incompetent, are presumed to be capable absent any evidence to the contrary.

The VA uses the term *mental competency* in a manner equivalent to SSA's use of *capability*, defining a mentally incompetent person as "one who because of injury or disease lacks the mental capacity to contract or to manage his or her own affairs, including disbursement of funds without limitation."[7] Adult beneficiaries are presumed to be competent to manage their own benefits unless there is clear and convincing evidence to the contrary (VA, 2015a). If there is a reasonable doubt[8] as to whether someone is capable of managing his or her own affairs, that doubt is resolved in favor of competency.[9]

---

[6] The information provided by AHIP that is presented in this chapter is based on a memorandum to the committee dated November 26, 2015, from Winthrop Cashdollar, Executive Director, Product Policy, AHIP (AHIP, 2015). This memorandum in its entirety is available in the committee's public access file.

[7] 38 CFR 3.353(a).

[8] Reasonable doubt means there is "an approximate balance of positive and negative evidence which does not satisfactorily prove or disprove the claim" (38 CFR 3.102).

[9] 38 CFR 3.353(d).

OPM (n.d.) uses the term *competency* in a similar manner, referring to an annuitant's mental or physical ability to handle his or her own benefits. Annuitants without a court-appointed fiduciary are presumed competent absent evidence to the contrary (Spear, 2015). Service Canada uses the term *capability* to describe those individuals suffering from severe mental impairment or a physical illness or impairment who are nonetheless able to manage their own affairs (Service Canada, 2015a).[10]

TRIGGERS FOR CAPABILITY ASSESSMENT

SSA provides the most in-depth information on potential triggers that bring capability into question during the disability determination process. When there is some indication or evidence that an adult SSDI or SSI beneficiary may not be able to manage or direct the management of his or her benefits and the beneficiary has not been judged legally incompetent, evidence of capability/incapability must be developed (i.e., gathered and evaluated). Two primary entities are involved in the disability determination process for an initial claim: the SSA field office and the state Disability Determination Service (DDS) agency. The field office is the first point of contact with the disability applicant, accepting applications for disability benefits and verifying nonmedical eligibility requirements. After this first step, the case is referred to the state DDS agency, where a disability examiner develops medical evidence and makes the initial determination of disability. Following that initial determination, the case is returned to the field office for appropriate action (e.g., nonmedical case development, computation of benefit amount, benefit payment). Either of these entities may identify the need to pursue capability case development.

Claims representatives at the SSA field offices are directed to develop evidence of capability when it is suspected that a mental or physical condition may inhibit the beneficiary's ability to manage or direct the management of his or her benefits (SSA, 2015e). In assessing whether development of evidence of capability is needed, claims representatives are instructed to consider two questions:

1. Does the individual have difficulty answering questions, getting the evidence or information necessary to pursue the claim, or understanding explanations and reporting instructions?

[10] Service Canada also uses the term *incapacity* with regard to persons who were or are incapable of forming or expressing an intention to make an application, to allow an application to be filed late in such circumstances. This is entirely separate from the issue of capability to manage benefits.

2. If so, do you think this difficulty indicates the beneficiary cannot manage or direct the management of funds?

In such cases, the field office forwards a request for capability case development to the state DDS agency along with the application for disability benefits. DDS is then responsible for providing an opinion regarding the claimant's capability to manage his or her disability benefits, along with medical evidence of disability. DDS also assumes this responsibility when its medical case development for determining whether a claimant has a disability indicates that a claimant may be incapable (SSA, 2015b).

SSA (2015c) operating instructions outline four situations for which medical evidence of capability must be developed by the disability examiner:

1. the field office indicates the claimant may be incapable and requests capability case development;
2. the claimant has a mental or physical impairment resulting in severe disorientation, a severe impairment of mental intellect, a gross deficit in judgment, or an inability to communicate with others;
3. a psychiatric or psychological consultative examination is purchased by the state DDS; or
4. someone other than the claimant filed the disability claim.

DDS disability examiners may develop evidence of capability in conjunction with the development of medical evidence of disability; DDS disability examiners do not complete medical case development solely to resolve capability issues. Box 2-1 provides information on training related to capability case development and determinations provided to field office and DDS staff.

For the VA, a beneficiary's competency is considered "whenever qualifying evidence raises a question as to the mental capacity to contract or to manage his/her own affairs, including disbursement of funds without limitation."[11] If the issue of competency is raised without supporting medical evidence or a statement from a responsible medical authority, additional medical evidence concerning competency must be developed.[12] (See the discussion of types and sources of evidence below.) The question of incompetency is raised if a beneficiary receives a 100 percent disability rating for a mental condition.[13] However, the 100 percent disability rating alone does not necessarily mean the person is unable to manage his or her benefits. For this reason, the VA regulations advise that such cases need to

[11] 38 CFR 3.353(a).
[12] 38 CFR 3.353(c).
[13] M21-1, Part III, Subpart IV, 8.A.2a.

BOX 2-1
Training in Capability Determinations for Field Office and Disability Determination Services (DDS) Staff

Field office claims representatives—nonmedical staff responsible for reviewing all evidence, adjudicating claims, and making the final determination regarding capability—are provided with all relevant program operations manual instructions on capability. Additionally, claims representatives complete an interactive video teletraining program that provides an overview of the representative payee program, including

- when a payee is needed,
- examples of the types of beneficiaries who may need a payee,
- how to conduct a capability determination,
- types of evidence (legal, medical, lay),
- guidance on how to select a suitable payee, and
- how to document the determination and payee selection.

DDS disability examiners—nonclinicians who receive 8-12 weeks of training in the SSA Listing of Impairments—collect and analyze medical evidence from the applicant's doctors and from hospitals, clinics, or institutions where the individual received treatment, as well as lay information about activities of daily living and work history. New examiners complete the Disability Examiner Basic Training Program (DEBT), which provides a comprehensive overview of the disability program, medical and vocational topics, case development processes, and case adjudication techniques. Among the lessons in DEBT, "Determine when and how to develop for capability" explains

- the overall capability policy;
- field office and DDS roles;
- when a capability opinion should be solicited;
- that medical case development should not be undertaken solely to resolve capability issues, but if any evidence raises capability issues, those issues should be resolved if possible; and
- how to annotate forms when capability is addressed.

SOURCES: Payne, 2015; Personal communication, M. Rochowiak, Office of Disability Policy, SSA, October 14, 2015.

be carefully considered to determine whether a proposal of incompetency is warranted.[14]

OPM generally identifies the need to determine competency in one of two ways. The first is through correspondence from someone familiar with

[14] 38 CFR 3.353.

the beneficiary (e.g., a family member, neighbor, or institution) suggesting that the annuitant is unable to manage his or her affairs. The second is through OPM's program integrity efforts, including surveys and matching. Information provided through a survey response may identify a potential need for representative payment and prompt further inquiry into this question. Likewise, if a survey is not returned or is returned as undeliverable, further inquiry is made as to why, which may lead to information that brings capability into question.

The regulations and functional guidance on third-party administration of benefits available to the committee contain no information on how potentially incapable beneficiaries may be identified in the Canadian system. The committee was told that Service Canada has no systematic approach for identifying such individuals; generally, such cases are brought to the attention of Service Canada by an individual who is familiar with the beneficiary, such as a family member, friend, or neighbor.

Private insurers reported a number of ways in which they identify claimants who may not be capable of managing their benefits. Potential triggers cited by respondents include a diagnosis (e.g., mental illness, behavioral health conditions, or brain injury that may impair cognitive functioning); a request for redirection of funds to a third party by someone familiar with the beneficiary (e.g., physician, family member); notification of a guardianship, conservatorship, power of attorney, or tutorship of the estate for the claimant; or personal interactions with the claimant that cause concern (e.g., confusion, engagement in risky behavior, or other signs of incompetence) (AHIP, 2015).

TYPES AND SOURCES OF EVIDENCE

SSA designates three categories of evidence in the capability determination process: legal, medical, and lay. To ensure consistency with SSA's language and allow for comparisons between SSA's capability determination process and that of other agencies and organizations, the committee discusses evidence of capability in accordance with this terminology. All of the programs reviewed rely on some combination of legal, medical, and lay evidence, although the primary evidence required for determining capability differs among organizations.

Legal Evidence

Legal evidence comprises findings regarding competence by the courts. SSA beneficiaries who have been declared legally incompetent through a court order are required to receive their funds through a representative payee. In such cases, the court's findings are reviewed and adopted as the determination of incapability, and no further development of evidence is required. It is important to note that what constitutes legal incompetence varies among states; therefore, as described below, the requirements for a finding of legal incompetence in some states may deviate from SSA's requirements for a finding of financial incapability.

SSA (2014b, 2015f) also notes that many states have moved away from specific findings of legal incompetence; in such cases, evidence of incompetence often takes the form of a court order appointing a legal guardian or conservator. If the court order does not specifically find the beneficiary legally incompetent or provide information about the individual's ability to manage financial affairs, SSA must clarify whether the order represents a finding of incompetence to manage financial affairs. In such cases, evaluators first consult the *Digest of State Guardianship Laws* to help determine whether the court order represents a finding of legal incompetence (SSA, 2015f). If incompetency still is not established by the court order, the court's findings may serve as evidence for the capability determination if they describe the beneficiary's ability or lack of ability to manage funds. However, further development of medical and lay evidence of capability is necessary (SSA, 2014b).

As with SSA, legal evidence may also be binding on OPM and Service Canada. An original or certified copy of a court order appointing a guardian, conservator, or fiduciary is sufficient for OPM to establish the need for a representative payee (OPM, 2013). For all other cases, medical and lay evidence is required. For Service Canada, when a legal arrangement is in place for another person or agency to act on the beneficiary's behalf, no further development or certification of capability is necessary. Such arrangements include an enduring power of attorney, public trustee, or court-appointed committee or guardian. These arrangements are binding and must be recognized, and CPP and/or OAS benefits must be paid directly to federally or provincially appointed administrators.

In contrast, a finding of legal incompetency by a court is not binding with respect to the competency of a veteran in the VA system.[15,16] However, such a legal finding does raise the question of competency, triggering the need to develop necessary medical evidence, and is to be given great weight in the VA process in conjunction with the medical evidence.[17] Evaluators are instructed to render an incompetency rating only when the evidence is clear and convincing and leaves no doubt as to the person's incompetency.[18] Court appointment of a fiduciary without a judicial determination of

[15] M21-1, Part III, Subpart IV, 8.A.1b.

[16] However, when a parent, surviving spouse, or adult helpless child is found incompetent by court decree, no further development of evidence is necessary (38 CFR 13.58).

[17] M21-1, Part III, Subpart IV, 8.A.5.b.

[18] 38 CFR 3.353.

incompetency or medical evidence is not considered evidence of incompetency requiring rating action.[19]

Medical Evidence

Medical evidence comprises information about a person's physical or mental condition (e.g., medical signs and laboratory findings, medical history and treatment records, opinions from medical sources) that sheds light on a beneficiary's ability to manage or direct the management of funds, based on an examination of the beneficiary by a medical professional. For SSA, such information must come "from a physician, psychologist or other qualified medical practitioner who is in a position to provide a meaningful assessment of the beneficiary's ability to manage funds" (SSA, 2012a). This may include a statement directly from the medical professional (e.g., on SSA Form 787, sent to the treating physician by the SSA field office), or other medical forms or summary reports from qualified medical professionals. Acceptable medical evidence must be based on an examination of the beneficiary performed within the last year. An opinion from a DDS agency that has reviewed the beneficiary's claim and medical evidence may provide evidence of incapability; it is not a determination of capability.

In weighing the value of medical evidence for determining capability, SSA notes the importance of using "good judgment":

> For example, a medical opinion of capability from a consultative examiner or another physician based on limited contact with the beneficiary is less convincing than an opinion from the treating source. Likewise, a medical opinion based on an examination of more than a year ago would not be as valuable as more recent evidence. (SSA, 2012a)

Although medical evidence is deemed "a very important consideration in determining a beneficiary's capability," it is not "definitive" for determining capability (SSA, 2012a). In contrast, the VA, OPM, and Service Canada require medical evidence to find a beneficiary incompetent.

According to the VA (2015a)[20] guidelines for evaluating competency, "a finding of incompetency cannot be made without a definite expression by a responsible medical authority unless the medical evidence of record is

- clear,
- convincing, and
- leaves no doubt as to the beneficiary's incompetency."

---

[19] 38 CFR 13.59.

[20] 38 CFR 3.353; M21-1, Part III, Subpart IV, 8.A.1d.

Medical evidence of competency is provided by an evaluating physician, and can range from a simple statement that the beneficiary cannot manage his or her funds to a detailed account of the person's functional incapacity. When the medical evidence is unclear, is unconvincing, or leaves doubt, additional medical evidence, which may include a VA examination to settle the question, must be developed before the case is forwarded to the rating activity.[21] If the individual is being seen or treated at a VA medical center or by a private care provider, the VBA will attempt to obtain those records as well (Flohr and Lewis, 2015).

For OPM, medical evidence must include a statement from a treating physician on his or her letterhead. Specific instructions, as discussed below, are provided to the treating physician as to the type of evidence required to make a competency determination.

Service Canada requires that for a beneficiary to be found incapable, he or she must be suffering from "severe mental impairment or a physical illness or impairment." Except in "exceptional circumstances," evidence of incapability must be submitted via a Certificate of Incapability (see Appendix C) by a *certified medical professional* (i.e., physician, registered nurse, nurse practitioner, psychologist, or psychiatrist). The medical professional certifying incapability must provide a diagnosis of the impairment, indicate in the appropriate box that he or she considers the individual to be incapable of managing his or her own affairs, and cite such incapability in the answer to at least one of five questions (as discussed below).

Private insurers reported that claims professionals will generally gather additional information by engaging the claimant's treating physician. However, they also reported that before attempting to gather additional information through conversations with potential informants or requests for medical evidence, they obtain legal authorization to do so.[22] Some insurers reported that a determination of incapability requires a definitive response by a treating physician to a specific question regarding capability; for these insurers, such a response is required regardless of how the issue was raised (AHIP, 2015).

Lay Evidence

Lay evidence comprises anything other than legal or medical evidence, as defined above, that provides material and relevant facts as to

[21] A "*rating activity* is a group of specially qualified employees vested with the authority to make decisions and take other actions on claims that require a rating decision," including competency (VA, 2015b).

[22] It is unclear from the information provided to the committee from whom this authorization is sought.

the beneficiary's ability to manage or direct the management of funds and meet his or her basic needs. Such evidence can be provided by anyone with direct knowledge of facts or circumstances regarding the beneficiary in his or her daily life; this may include nonprofessionals (e.g., relatives, friends, neighbors) and health care and other professionals (e.g., social workers, occupational therapists, rehabilitation specialists, adult protective services workers).

To find a beneficiary incapable, SSA requires lay evidence. It considers such evidence to be "anything other than legal or medical evidence, which gives insight into a beneficiary's ability to manage or direct the management of his/her funds" to meet daily needs (i.e., food, shelter, clothing). For SSA, this evidence may include direct observations of the beneficiary's behavior, reasoning ability, and functioning; statements from or contact with third parties, such as relatives, friends, neighbors, landlords, representatives of community groups, or professionals who do not provide "evidence of a medical nature"[23] (e.g., social workers, occupational therapists, caseworkers, rehabilitation counselors, clergy); and a representative payee applicant's answer to why the applicant thinks the claimant is unable to handle his or her affairs (SSA, 2011a).[24] SSA notes that a face-to-face interview with the beneficiary, when possible, is "the best source for lay evidence of capability" because it provides "the opportunity to observe the beneficiary's behavior, ability to reason, ability to function with others, and effectiveness with which he [or] she pursues the claim" (SSA, 2011b).

OPM also requires lay evidence for determining a beneficiary's competency. Acceptable lay evidence takes the form of sworn affidavits from persons (preferably one family member and one non-family member) who know the beneficiary and facts concerning his or her competency.

For the VA, lay evidence may be considered following an initial determination of incompetency. For example, "after development of information with regard to social, economic, and industrial adjustment, the Veterans Service Center Manager may be of the opinion that a beneficiary rated, or proposed to be rated, incompetent is actually capable of handling, without limitation, the funds payable." Such evidence is then referred back to the

---

[23] SSA defines evidence of a medical nature as evidence "from a physician, psychologist or other qualified medical practitioner who is in a position to provide a meaningful assessment of the beneficiary's ability to manage funds." All other nonlegal evidence, from other professionals and lay persons familiar with the beneficiary, is considered lay evidence.

[24] Relevant forms include *Request to Be Selected as Payee* (Form SSA-11-BK), *Function Report—Adult* (Form SSA-3373-BK), and *Function Report—Adult—Third Party* (Form SSA-3380-BK). The first asks why the applicant thinks the claimant is unable to handle his or her own benefits, and the latter two include questions about the individual's ability to handle money, as well as other activities of daily living. See Appendix C for these forms.

VA rating activity for consideration of all the evidence.[25] The beneficiary and any witnesses of his or her choice may also provide lay evidence at a personal hearing following notification of plans to appoint a fiduciary.[26]

Service Canada likewise may rely on lay evidence of incapability, which it collects via the Certificate of Incapability (as outlined above for collecting medical evidence). Service Canada allows for this evidence to be submitted by a nonmedical professional (i.e., a lawyer, social worker, or member of the clergy) in "exceptional circumstances," such as for beneficiaries living in remote locations or vulnerable seniors who are homeless or at imminent risk of being homeless; incapability cannot be certified by nonprofessionals (Service Canada, 2015b) (see Table 2-3 for a list of acceptable professionals). Meeting these requirements, the certificate will serve as acceptable evidence of the beneficiary's incapability. Regardless of whether the form is submitted by a medical or nonmedical professional, the information thus provided may fit the committee's definition of lay evidence.

Private insurers reported that claims professionals will gather information on capability by engaging members of the claimant's family on whom he or she relies extensively (AHIP, 2015).

INSTRUCTIONS TO INFORMANTS

Instructions to informants vary widely among programs. SSA operating instructions provide an extensive list of recommended questions for field office staff conducting face-to-face interviews, but no such information is provided to medical professionals or persons providing lay evidence of capability. The form provided to the treating physician by the SSA field office (SSA-787; see Appendix C) provides little guidance on the basis for an opinion on capability, asking:

> Do you believe the patient is capable of managing or directing the management of benefits in his or her own best interest? By capable we mean that the patient:
> - Is able to understand and act on the ordinary affairs of life, such as providing for own adequate food, housing, clothing, etc., and
> - Is able, in spite of physical impairments, to manage funds or direct others how to manage them.

In contrast, OPM provides the most in-depth instructions on the type of information necessary to make a determination of capability. OPM Form RI 30-3 (see Appendix C), to be used by physicians and persons providing

[25] 38 CFR 3.353(b)(3).
[26] M21-1, Part III, Subpart IV, 9.B.6.

TABLE 2-3 Persons Qualified to Complete the Certificate of Incapability for Service Canada

Standard Third-Party Administration	In Exceptional Circumstances (e.g., remote locations)	For Homeless Seniors
Certified medical professional • Physician (preferred) • Registered nurse • Nurse practitioner • Psychologist • Psychiatrist	Certified medical professional • Physician (preferred) • Registered nurse • Nurse practitioner • Psychologist • Psychiatrist	Certified medical professional • Physician (preferred) • Registered nurse • Nurse practitioner • Psychologist • Psychiatrist
	or	or
	Lawyer who has been handling the person's affairs Social worker Member of the clergy	Lawyer Social worker

SOURCE: Service Canada, 2015b, p. 30.

lay evidence, outlines the specific information necessary for a competency determination (OPM, 2013). Physicians are instructed to provide a "history of the specific medical condition(s) which caused the individual to be incompetent, including symptoms, physical findings, results of laboratory studies, and therapy (together with the response to therapy)," as well as the duration of the condition causing incompetency and the expected date of full or partial recovery. In addition to this statement, physicians are asked to provide copies of all relevant laboratory reports, psychological test reports, and discharge summaries of hospitalizations. For informants providing lay evidence, OPM Form RI 30-3 specifies that affidavits should provide information on the individual's relationship to and amount of contact with the beneficiary, observed actions or incidents that call the beneficiary's competency to manage his or her affairs into question, reasons why there is no court-appointed guardian or fiduciary, and information on who has been handling the individual's affairs (OPM, 2013; Spear, 2015).

Service Canada also asks specific questions of medical (or in rare cases, nonmedical) professionals regarding capability. Informants certifying capability must provide a diagnosis (if a medical professional) or description (if a nonmedical professional) of the impairment, indicate in the appropriate box that he or she considers the individual to be incapable of managing his or her own affairs, and cite such incapability in the answer to at least one of the following questions:

- Does the person named above have good general knowledge of what is happening to his/her money or investments?
- Does the person named above have sufficient understanding of the concept of time, in order to pay bills promptly?
- Does the person named above have sufficient memory to keep track of financial transactions and decisions?
- Does the person named above have ability to balance accounts and bills?
- Does the person named above have significant impairment of judgment due to altered intellectual function?

It is unclear whether the VA provides any formal guidance to potential informants.

DEVELOPING EVIDENCE AND DETERMINING CAPABILITY

Social Security Administration

SSA field offices and state DDS agencies both play a role in developing evidence of capability. DDS disability examiners are responsible for requesting medical records from all sources listed on the disability application and developing all medical evidence for a disability claim. The primary role of the DDS agency is to review the medical evidence to make an initial determination regarding disability; however, it is alert for any indication or statement from a medical provider regarding an applicant's ability to manage funds (Payne, 2015). When a medical professional specifically offers an opinion on capability, the DDS agency needs to pursue no further development of medical evidence in reference to the capability issue (SSA, 2015b). Such an opinion may be included in a summary statement from the treating medical professional. Additionally, any time a psychological or psychiatric consultative examination is purchased to assess disability, the consultative examiner (a medical professional) is asked to provide a statement on capability (SSA, 2015b).

The DDS agency also may provide an opinion on capability, based on all available evidence. If evidence from an acceptable medical source is available, the DDS agency may categorize the question as "resolved" and offer its opinion on the beneficiary's capability. When such evidence is not available, the DDS agency may still provide an opinion based on third-party sources, but will report the question of capability as "unresolved" (SSA, 2014a). At this point, the DDS agency will remit its opinion on capability, along with supporting evidence, to the field office, where the responsibility for rendering a definitive judgment of capability resides.

As noted above, although medical evidence is important and informative for SSA in determining capability, it is not definitive; lay evidence is requisite for all SSA capability determinations. Whereas the primary role of the DDS agency is to evaluate medical evidence, the field office claims representative is trained to adjudicate all nonmedical factors in a disability claim. The DDS agency's opinion on capability serves as evidence, to be weighed along with all other available evidence. In evaluating whether a beneficiary is capable, the claims representative develops lay evidence, weighs all available evidence, and makes a determination on capability.[27]

Claims representatives are instructed to "obtain as much lay evidence as [they] consider necessary to make a reasoned capability determination [and] use [their] judgment to determine how much lay evidence is needed to make the correct capability determination" (SSA, 2011b). Such evidence may be acquired in a number of ways. As noted above, SSA operating instructions state that face-to-face interviews are the best source for lay evidence of capability, and claims representatives are given a list of sample questions (SSA, 2011b) (see Box 2-2). Data provided to the committee for fiscal year 2013 show that a large majority of SSDI claims are awarded without the beneficiary's visiting the field office (i.e., with no face-to-face contact) (see Table 2-4). As noted, lay evidence also may be obtained through statements from third parties familiar with the beneficiary (e.g., friends, relatives, social workers, and any community service groups with which he or she has contact) about how the person manages money. When evidence is deemed insufficient to make a determination, field visits to the beneficiary's home for observation may be considered (SSA, 2011b), but information is not available on how frequently this occurs.

Upon determination that a beneficiary is incapable, SSA provides advance notice to the beneficiary before appointing the payee. This notice must inform the beneficiary that SSA has determined he or she needs a representative payee; provide the name of the proposed representative payee; and state the beneficiary's appeal rights, including the right to appeal the determination or the designation of a particular person, review the evidence

[27] As noted in Chapter 1, the scope of the present study is limited to disability beneficiaries. For this population, a determination of whether an individual is capable is made only once the individual has been determined to be eligible for disability benefits; therefore, a disability determination is assumed. As evidence of capability is developed during the initial determination stage, the discussion of SSA's process for determining financial capability focuses primarily on the SSA field office and the state DDS agency. However, it is important to note here that some individuals are determined to have a disability following appeal of the initial disability determination. During the appeals process, an opinion on capability may be provided by an entity other than the SSA field office or the state DDS agency, such as an administrative law judge (ALJ). However, unless the question of capability is specifically set before the ALJ, this opinion is to be treated as lay evidence and considered along with all other evidence. The field office is responsible for making the final determination (SSA, 2012b).

BOX 2-2
Sample Capability Assessment Questions for the SSA Field Office Claims Representatives

Financial Management

The answers to these questions will likely demonstrate self-awareness and the ability to address current needs, the beneficiary's understanding of the value of money, the beneficiary's independence and self-sufficiency, and the ability to handle problems.

- What bills do you have to pay each month? Or When you live on your own, what bills will you have to pay? (Rent? Utilities? Food? Transportation?)
- Do you pay these bills (i.e., rent/mortgage, utilities, etc.) or does someone else pay them for you?
- Do you ever forget to pay some bills?
- If you ever forgot to pay a bill, what did you do about it? How did you find out about it?
- Can you make change?
- Do you ever go to the bank? If yes, how often?
- Do you have a bank account? If yes, is it a checking or savings account? If it is a checking account, do you write the checks? If not, does someone else write checks on your account?
- If you have a checking account, did you ever write a check for insufficient funds ("bounced" a check)? How often has this happened? Why do you think this happened and what did you do about it when it happened?
- If you have a bank account, how often do you get a statement from the bank? What do you do with the statement? Do you read and understand it?
- What are the most important things to spend money on?

Shelter

The following questions provide essential information in determining the ability to meet basic daily needs, stability in living arrangements, and existing support network.

- In what type of housing do you live?
- How long have you lived there? If less than 1 year, where did you live before?
- Do you live alone? If not, who lives with you?

Food

Quality/nutritional value of food could be a significant clue regarding ability to meet basic daily needs. Assistance in these tasks could be significant regarding support network/independence.

- How many meals per day do you usually eat? What kind of food do you usually eat?

- Do you ever go to the store to buy groceries? If not, does anyone else buy groceries for you? Who?
- Do you decide what groceries you need to buy? If not, who decides?
- If you go to the store to buy groceries, how do you get there?
- If you ran out of food before your check came, what would you do?

Medical

The following questions could provide essential information regarding the beneficiary's ability to meet basic medical needs.

- Do you ever see a doctor? If so, where do you go and how often? If not, why not?
- Do you take medication? If yes, do you need help remembering when and how much to take?
- How do you pay the doctor's bill or pay for medicine?

Support Network

The following questions attempt to provide a measure of insight into the beneficiary's existing family, friends, or acquaintances who can be counted on to help.

- Do you have any relatives who live nearby?
- Do you have any friends or other people you can trust?
- Do your friends or relatives help you in any way? Do you ask your friends or relatives for help when you need it?
- Is there a community center or other group that helps you or teaches you how to budget your money and pay your bills each month?
- Do your friends or family help you figure out how to manage your funds?

General

The following questions could provide insight into the beneficiary's thought processes, ability to reason, value system, etc., and could give clues regarding a beneficiary's vulnerability to predators.

- What things besides food do you shop for each month?
- Do friends or family ever borrow money from you and not pay you back?
- Do people ever borrow things you own and not give them back?
- Have you ever lived with people that did not pay their share of the rent or other expenses?
- If, in the last year, you have lived with friends or family, did they charge you for the rent? If yes, how much?

SOURCE: SSA, 2011b.

TABLE 2-4 Social Security Disability Insurance (SSDI) Claims by Representative Payee Status and Type of Contact Between Beneficiary and Field Office Staff

SSDI Claims	Office Visit	No Office Visit	Total
With representative payee	23,858	34,565	58,423
Without representative payee	185,841	400,795	586,636
Total	209,699	435,360	645,059

SOURCE: Personal communication, M. Rochowiak, Office of Disability Policy, SSA, October 14, 2015.

on which the decision is based, and submit additional information (SSA, 2011c; 42 USC 405 § 205).

U.S. Department of Veterans Affairs

When a regional office receives credible evidence that indicates a beneficiary may be unable to manage his or her affairs, the evidence is sent to a VA rating activity, which is responsible for making the original competency decision (VA, 2015b). The Rating Veterans Service Representative (RVSR)[28] or a designee is responsible for proposing initial competency determinations based on clear and convincing medical evidence (VA, 2015a). As noted above, if the medical evidence is unclear or unconvincing (i.e., is insufficient to make a competency determination), a Veterans Service Representative (VSR) develops additional evidence, including by scheduling an exam to help make the determination (Flohr and Lewis, 2015; VA, 2015a). If, after further evidence development, there still is not clear and convincing medical evidence of incompetency (i.e., there is reasonable doubt), the beneficiary is presumed competent.[29] If the evidence only *suggests* that the beneficiary is incapable, the case is not developed, nor is a proposal of incompetency made, and the rating decision must state that there was no clear and convincing evidence of incompetency (VA, 2015a). If there is clear and convincing evidence that a beneficiary is incapable of managing his or her VA benefits without limitation, the rating activity proposes an incompetency rating (Flohr and Lewis, 2015).

[28] RSVRs come from a variety of backgrounds, including veterans, attorneys, and nurses. They receive 6 weeks of intensive training at a central location upon being hired, followed by additional training at the regional office. RSVRs also are required to complete 60 hours of training per year (Flohr and Lewis, 2015).

[29] 38 CFR 3.353.

If the rating activity proposes an incompetency rating, the VSR or designee provides the beneficiary with a copy of the proposed incompetency rating or a summary of the evidence supporting the finding of incompetency; an explanation of the effect of the finding on the payment of the VA benefits; and notice that a VA rating of incompetency prevents the beneficiary from purchasing firearms, according to the Brady Handgun Violence Prevention Act (the Brady Act) (VA, 2015a,c). In addition, the beneficiary is notified of his or her appeal rights, including the opportunity to submit additional evidence and to appear at a hearing with representation, if desired, and informed that he or she has 60 days to respond to the notice.[30,31] Sample language for a VA notice of a proposed rating of incompetency to a beneficiary, as provided in the VBA's adjudication procedures, is presented in Box 2-3. The VSR also sends notice of the initial incompetency determination, including the evidence upon which it is based, to the appropriate fiduciary hub with a request for appointment of a fiduciary, custodian, or guardian (Flohr and Lewis, 2015; VA, 2015a).

If no additional evidence or request for a hearing is filed during the due process period, jurisdiction of the proposed decision is transferred to a fiduciary service representative at the fiduciary hub,[32] who has the authority to finalize the proposed determination of incompetency (VA, 2015a). After finalizing the incompetency determination, the fiduciary hub takes action to appoint a fiduciary, generally within 45 days, by conducting a face-to-face visit with the beneficiary and proposed fiduciary. The appointment process includes an investigation of the evidence that supports the beneficiary's incompetency to manage funds and the qualifications of the proposed fiduciary. After considering the evidence compiled during the appointment process, the fiduciary hub may (1) concur with the incompetency determination and appoint a fiduciary; (2) conclude that the beneficiary is incompetent, but able to manage VA benefits with supervision (supervised direct payment); or (3) disagree with the incompetency determination and remit the case to the rating activity with evidence that supports this opinion. For cases in which the fiduciary hub disagrees with the incompetency rating, the appointment of the fiduciary is confirmed, and the fiduciary receives VA benefits on behalf of the beneficiary while the rating activity again considers the issue of competency (Flohr and Lewis, 2015; VA, 2015c).

Under the supervised direct payment option, "benefits payable to a veteran rated incompetent may be paid directly to the veteran in such

---

[30] 38 CFR 3.103.

[31] A due process notice is not required if the beneficiary is determined to be incompetent by a court of competent jurisdiction.

[32] The VA fiduciary operations are consolidated into six regional "hubs," which provide oversight of the VA's fiduciary program.

BOX 2-3
Sample Language for a Notice of a Proposed Rating of Incompetency

We have received information showing that because of your disabilities you may need help in handling your U.S. Department of Veterans Affairs (VA) benefits. We received the information from [**name of physician, medical institution, etc.**]. The report, dated [**date of the report**], shows [**brief description of the diagnosis and/or findings**].

We must decide if you are able to handle your VA benefit payments. We will base our decision on all the evidence we already have and any other evidence you may wish to send us. Before we make a final determination, you have the right to submit any evidence, information, or statement that will present your side of the case.

What We Propose to Do

We propose to rate you incompetent for the VA purposes. This means a fiduciary may be appointed to help you manage your VA benefits. Payment of any money due you will be made directly to your fiduciary. This person or institution must use your payments for your benefit and is responsible to the VA for their use.

We have enclosed a copy of our Rating Decision for your review. It provides a detailed explanation about our proposal, the reason for it, and the evidence considered.

When and Where to Send the Information or Evidence

Please mail or fax all responses to the appropriate address listed on the attached Where to Send Your Written Correspondence chart within **60 days** from the date of this letter. Please put your full name and the VA file number on the evidence. If we do not receive the information or evidence within that time, we will make our decision based only on the evidence we have received.

How This Decision Could Affect You

A determination of incompetency will prohibit you from purchasing, possessing, receiving, or transporting a firearm or ammunition. If you knowingly violate any

amount as the Veterans Service Center Manager determines the veteran is able to manage with continuing supervision by the Veterans Service Center Manager, provided a fiduciary is not otherwise required."[33] This option provides the beneficiary with greater autonomy in managing his or her benefits, and allows for an assessment of the beneficiary's performance

[33] 38 CFR 13.56.

prohibition, pursuant to section 924(a)(2) of title 18, United States Code (USC), as implemented by Public Law 103-159 of the Brady Handgun Violence Prevention Act, you may be fined, imprisoned, or both.

If we decide that you are unable to handle your VA funds, you may apply to the VA for the relief of prohibitions imposed by the Brady Act with regards to the possession, purchase, receipt, or transportation of a firearm. Submit your request on the enclosed VA Form 21-4138, Statement in Support of Claim. The VA will determine whether such relief is warranted.

How to Obtain a Personal Hearing

If you desire a personal hearing to present evidence or argument about your ability to handle your VA benefits, notify this office and we will arrange a time and place for the hearing. If you want, you may bring witnesses and their testimony will be entered in the record. The VA will furnish the hearing room and provide hearing officials. The VA cannot pay any other expenses of the hearing because a personal hearing is held only on your request.

Please notify us as soon as possible if you would like to request a hearing. If the VA receives your hearing request prior to the final competency determination, we will continue to send payments to you until we have held the hearing and reviewed the testimony. If no request for hearing is received prior to the final competency determination, a decision will be made based on the evidence of record.

How to Obtain Representation

An accredited representative of a veterans' organization or other service organization recognized by the Secretary of Veterans Affairs may represent you, without charge. An accredited agent or attorney may also represent you. However, under 38 USC 5904(c), an accredited agent or attorney may only charge you for services performed after the date you file a notice of disagreement. If you desire representation, let us know and we will send you the necessary forms. If you have already designated a representative, no further action is required on your part.

within the first year and reassessment of the incompetency rating based on this information.

Office of Personnel Management

Depending on the complexity of the case, a customer specialist (GS-7), junior legal administrative specialist (GS-5 to GS-11), or senior legal administrative specialist (GS-12)[34] handles issues relating to competency. A customer specialist handles routine issues, such as cases for which there is a court order establishing that a representative payee is needed. For less clear-cut cases, a legal administrative specialist seeks out and assesses the necessary medical and lay evidence to make a decision concerning competency. A physician under contract to OPM also is available to legal administrative specialists if questions about the medical condition arise. Legal administrative specialists must complete 1 year of formal training with a concentration in medical conditions and terminology; additional training is provided on process flow and preparation of letters (Spear, 2015).

The process for establishing incompetency and assigning a representative payee can take anywhere from 30 to 90 days, depending on complicating factors or the need for additional inquiry or investigation. Upon determination of incompetency, OPM notifies the annuitant or the survivor annuitant that a representative payee has been designated (Spear, 2015).

Service Canada

If it meets the requirements outlined above, the Certificate of Incapability will serve as acceptable evidence of a beneficiary's incapability. The certificate is then reviewed by a Service Canada benefits officer, answers to the questions and any commentary are assessed, and the signatory is verified, at which point a trustee is generally appointed. In rare situations, however, the case may be referred to CPP medical professionals for additional assessment (Kidd, 2015).

APPEALS PROCESSES

With the exception of Service Canada, all of the programs examined have official appeals processes, with SSA's process being the most in-depth, allowing for multiple levels of appeal. An SSA incapability determination may first be appealed through an informal *protest* or a formal *request for reconsideration*. To be considered a formal request, the appeal must be in writing, made by the beneficiary or a person who can act for the beneficiary, and in response to an initial determination. The beneficiary has 60 days to request an appeal. If a protest or request for reconsideration is received

[34] The majority of federal government employee positions are graded on the General Schedule (GS), from GS-1 to GS-15, which is the highest attainable level. Most entry-level positions are between GS-5 and GS-7, and mid-level positions range from GS-8 to GS-12. GS-4 specialists require 1 year of general experience and at least 2 years of credits after high school. GS-5 specialists require at least 1 year of specialized experience equivalent to GS-4. Four years of credits after high school is required to attain the GS-5 level. Any GS level higher than 5 requires specialized experience of at least the grade level below.

before the payee has been appointed (generally within 10 days of the beneficiary's receipt of the notification), the appointment will not take effect until the appeal has been resolved; if a case cannot be resolved immediately, direct payment will be made to the beneficiary, if possible, until the case is resolved (SSA, 2012c). If the determination is protested after the 10-day period, payment to the representative payee will begin.

When an incapability determination is appealed, the decision is first reviewed by a claims representative who was not involved in the original decision. Any new information provided by the beneficiary, or someone acting on his or her behalf, is reviewed along with the existing evidence. A face-to-face interview with the beneficiary may be requested to resolve any problems. If the beneficiary is deemed capable, direct payment begins immediately. If the selection of the representative payee was appealed and a new payee is selected, the beneficiary is given advance notice of the revised selection and allowed time to appeal it (SSA, 2012c). If the initial determination is upheld in reconsideration, the beneficiary may accept the decision or exercise his or her right to an appeal before an administrative law judge (SSA, 2006). Data from SSA on the number of beneficiaries who appeal a capability determination were unavailable to the committee.

As with SSA, a VA beneficiary has 60 days to respond in writing to the notice of a proposed rating of incompetency if he or she chooses to appeal the rating.[35,36] If additional evidence or a hearing request is received, the RSVR at the rating office that is collocated with the fiduciary hub has jurisdiction to make the final determination (VA, 2015a). The RSVR conducts all requested hearings, reviews all additional medical evidence submitted, and renders the final decision regarding competency.

OPM provides its beneficiaries the opportunity to appeal within 10 days of the decision, during which time the beneficiary may provide additional evidence for review by the contract doctor. If the beneficiary is still found incompetent, he or she may further appeal to the Merit Systems Protection Board.

Unlike SSA, the VA, and OPM, Service Canada has no formal appeals process for individuals who are deemed incapable, as "any decision by the Department regarding an appointment of a trustee for the purposes of administering CPP and/or OAS benefits is made under the Minister's discretion and is therefore not appealable" (Service Canada, 2015b, p. 13).

No private insurers identified a formal appeals process.

---

[35] 38 CFR 3.102.

[36] A due process notice is not required if the beneficiary is determined to be incompetent by a court of competent jurisdiction.

REVIEW

None of the programs examined have a formal process for ongoing review of all beneficiaries (regardless of whether the beneficiary was initially found capable or incapable). However, each program defines specific instances that may warrant considering such a review.

For SSA, the issue of capability may be reevaluated whenever there is some indication or evidence that an incapable beneficiary has become capable or a previously capable beneficiary now may be incapable. Claims representatives are instructed to "consider reviewing" capability in such cases by "examining the indicators in a case and deciding whether full development is needed" (SSA, 2015e). Specific situations that require such a review include continuing disability reviews (CDRs),[37] SSI redeterminations, discovery that an incapable beneficiary manages any other benefits, beneficiary appeal, or any other contact with the beneficiary that raises the question of his or her capability (SSA, 2015e). It is not known how many beneficiaries with representative payees are determined to need a payee at the time of the initial determination versus some later time, as SSA does not collect data that differentiate new appointments from change-of-payee actions.[38]

The VA has a process for reviewing beneficiaries who have previously been rated incompetent. The VA field examiners contact incompetent beneficiaries every 1 to 3 years to review both their incompetence ratings and their fiduciaries' performance (Flohr and Lewis, 2015). The majority of these contacts occur through face-to-face visits with the beneficiary, but contact may take place by telephone or letter when a beneficiary is in a protected environment licensed by a state or local government and the beneficiary's benefit is below a prescribed threshold. Additionally, a beneficiary's competency can be reviewed any time new medical evidence is received. This may include evidence from a hospital summary, a report of release to or discharge from nonresidential care, or a report of some other material change in condition. Any such evidence that may call the previous rating into question is referred to the rating activity for review. The rating activity then considers this new evidence along with all other evidence to determine the beneficiary's current competency status.[39]

---

[37] By law, SSA is required to conduct a periodic medical CDR to determine whether an individual receiving disability benefits remains eligible to receive benefits. The prescribed interval between CDRs is 6-18 months when improvement is expected, up to 3 years when improvement is possible, and 5-7 years when improvement is not expected. Although in principle CDRs would provide a regular opportunity to review the beneficiary's capability status, as of the end of fiscal year 2013, there was a backlog of 1.3 million medical CDRs.

[38] Personal communication, M. Rochowiak, Office of Disability Policy, SSA, October 14, 2015.

[39] 38 CFR 3.353(b)(3).

OPM administers a representative payee survey every 2 years to ensure that federal retirement benefits are being expended for the benefit of the annuitant. One question—"Did you turn over any of the annuity benefits to another person during the survey period?"—may provide information about whether any of the annuity was given to the beneficiary so he or she could decide how to use the money (as noted in the OPM instructions for this question). This information may trigger further inquiry, which in turn may lead to reevaluation of the competency decision.

Service Canada allows for review of cases in certain situations. Professionals filling out the Certificate of Incapability are asked whether improvement is expected, and Service Canada staff, upon initial appointment of a trustee, "must establish whether the case should be reviewed at a later date in order to determine if the condition of the beneficiary has improved to the extent that the trusteeship should be terminated" (Service Canada, 2015b, p. 20). Cases may also be reviewed when a beneficiary informs Service Canada that he or she has regained capability; in such cases, Service Canada will require the trustee to provide a new Certificate of Incapability to substantiate or refute the claim. The trustee may also notify Service Canada if the beneficiary regains capability, in which case payments will be made directly to the beneficiary.

Although no private insurers provided information regarding their process for review of cases to identify changes in competency, information provided by AHIP indicated that such review is required periodically.

SUMMARY

The committee identified a number of points for comparison of the programs reviewed in this chapter, including the overall size of the program, the number of beneficiaries deemed incapable (or comparable determination), potential triggers for capability assessment, types of evidence considered, instructions to informants, appeals processes, and review processes. SSA's programs, both overall and with respect to the number of beneficiaries determined incapable, are significantly larger than all of the other programs examined by the committee.

Among the programs reviewed, SSA guidance provides the most in-depth information on potential triggers that call capability into question. However, a unique aspect of the OPM program in this regard is its use of computerized matching; although such matching is primarily for analysis of benefit disbursement from other programs that may impact OPM benefits, it may also provide information that brings capability into question.

All of the programs reviewed rely on some combination of legal, medical, and lay evidence, although the primary evidence relied upon for determining capability differs among organizations. SSA, OPM, and Service

Canada all conform to judicial findings of incompetence in some respect, while the VA considers such orders as nonbinding legal evidence to be considered along with all other evidence (however, the VA does consider a finding of legal incompetence to be a trigger for further examination of capability). The VA requires medical evidence; SSA requires lay evidence; OPM requires both medical and lay evidence (i.e., a statement from a treating physician and two affidavits from persons familiar with the beneficiary); and except in rare cases, Service Canada requires evidence from a medical professional via the Certificate of Incapability, which requests information both of a medical nature and on financial competence and performance. Instructions to informants on the information required to make a capability determination vary widely among programs. OPM provides both medical and lay evidence sources with robust guidance on the information needed to make a decision on capability via *Information Necessary for a Competency Determination* (see Appendix C). Service Canada also asks specific questions of medical (or in rare cases nonmedical) professionals regarding capability. SSA operating instructions provide an extensive list of recommended questions for field office staff conducting face-to-face interviews, but no such information is provided to medical professionals or persons providing lay evidence of capability. It is unclear whether the VA provides any formal guidance to potential informants.

Although SSA recognizes that face-to-face interviews are the best means of collecting lay evidence, decisions can be, and often are, made without direct interaction with the beneficiary. In contrast, the VA, with limited exceptions, meets face-to-face with every beneficiary who has been rated incompetent.

The VA provides two options for beneficiaries rated incompetent: appointment of a fiduciary and supervised direct pay. Supervised direct pay allows payment of benefits directly to certain high-functioning beneficiaries who have been rated incompetent. The option of supervised direct payment provides the beneficiary with greater autonomy in managing his or her benefits, and allows for an assessment of the beneficiary's performance within the first year and reassessment of the incompetency rating based on this information.

With the exception of Service Canada, all of the programs examined have official appeals processes, with SSA's process being the most in-depth, allowing for multiple levels of appeal. None of the programs examined have a formal process for ongoing review of all beneficiaries (regardless of whether the beneficiary was initially found capable or incapable); however, each program defines specific instances that may warrant considering such a review. The VA has a process for reviewing beneficiaries who have previously been rated incompetent. SSA may consider reviewing capability based on information obtained from a CDR, SSI redetermination, or beneficiary appeal; any other contact with the beneficiary that raises the question of his or her capability; or discovery that an incapable beneficiary manages any other benefits.

REFERENCES

AHIP (America's Health Insurance Plans). 2015. *Overview of private disability income protection insurer capability determination processes.* Washington, DC: AHIP.

Flohr, B., and C. Lewis. 2015. Veterans Benefits Administration incompetency determinations. Presentation to the Committee to Evaluate the Social Security Administration's Capability Determination Process for Adult Beneficiaries, April 21, Washington, DC.

Kidd, M. A. 2015. Canada Pension Plan and Old Age Security Program. Presentation to the Committee to Evaluate the Social Security Administration's Capability Determination Process for Adult Beneficiaries, October 9, Washington, DC.

OPM (U.S. Office of Personnel Management). 2013. *Information necessary for a competency determination.* Document RI 30-3. OMB Form number 3206-0140. Washington, DC: OPM.

OPM. n.d. *Representative payees.* https://www.opm.gov/retirement-services/my-annuity-and-benefits/representative-payees (accessed January 21, 2016).

Payne, D. 2015. Description of the Disability Determination Services' role in the capability determination process. Presentation to the Committee to Evaluate the Social Security Administration's Capability Determination Process for Adult Beneficiaries, February 3, Washington, DC.

Service Canada. 2015a. *Certificate of incapability.* Form SC ISP-3505. http://www.servicecanada.gc.ca/eforms/forms/sc-isp-3505(2015-07-03)e_cpp.pdf (accessed January 29, 2016).

Service Canada. 2015b. *Third party administration (functional guidance).* Ottawa, ON: Service Canada.

Spear, Q. 2015. OPM retirement program: Process for evaluating financial capability. Presentation to the Committee to Evaluate the Social Security Administration's Capability Determination Process for Adult Beneficiaries, June 24, Washington, DC.

SSA (U.S. Social Security Administration). 2003. *GN 00502.010 Capability determination—overview.* https://secure.ssa.gov/poms.nsf/lnx/0200502010 (accessed December 15, 2015).

SSA. 2006. *NL 00703.215 Notice affirming selection of representative payee on reconsideration.* https://secure.ssa.gov/apps10/poms.nsf/lnx/0900703215 (accessed December 15, 2015).

SSA. 2011a. *GN 00502.030 Lay evidence of capability.* https://secure.ssa.gov/apps10/poms.nsf/lnx/0200502030 (accessed December 15, 2015).

SSA. 2011b. *GN 00502.050 Developing evidence of capability.* https://secure.ssa.gov/poms.nsf/lnx/0200502050#a (accessed December 15, 2015).

SSA. 2011c. *GN 00503.110 Appeal rights.* https://secure.ssa.gov/apps10/poms.nsf/lnx/0200503110 (accessed December 15, 2015).

SSA. 2012a. *GN 00502.025 Medical evidence of capability.* https://secure.ssa.gov/apps10/poms.nsf/lnx/0200502025 (accessed December 15, 2015).

SSA. 2012b. *GN 00502.060 Making a capability determination.* https://secure.ssa.gov/poms.nsf/lnx/0200502060 (accessed January 28, 2016).

SSA. 2012c. *GN 00503.120 Response received to advance notice.* https://secure.ssa.gov/apps10/poms.nsf/lnx/0200503120 (accessed December 15, 2015).

SSA. 2014a. *DI 23001.015 Disability Determination Services (DDS) procedures for documenting capability*. https://secure.ssa.gov/apps10/poms.nsf/lnx/0423001015 (accessed December 15, 2015).

SSA. 2014b. *GN 00502.005 Direct payment prohibitions*. https://secure.ssa.gov/apps10/poms.nsf/lnx/0200502005 (accessed December 15, 2015).

SSA. 2015a. *Annual statistical supplement*. https://www.socialsecurity.gov/policy/docs/statcomps/supplement/2015/index.html (accessed February 8, 2016).

SSA. 2015b. *DI 23001.001 Disability Determination Services (DDS) capability opinion*. https://secure.ssa.gov/apps10/poms.nsf/lnx/0423001001 (accessed December 15, 2015).

SSA. 2015c. *DI 23001.005 Disability Determination Services (DDS) procedures for determining capability*. https://secure.ssa.gov/apps10/poms.nsf/lnx/0423001005 (accessed December 15, 2015).

SSA. 2015d. *Fast facts and figures about Social Security, 2015*. https://www.socialsecurity.gov/policy/docs/chartbooks/fast_facts/2015/fast_facts15.pdf (accessed January 24, 2016).

SSA. 2015e. *GN 00502.020 Determining capability—adult beneficiaries*. https://secure.ssa.gov/poms.nsf/lnx/0200502020 (accessed December 15, 2015).

SSA. 2015f. *GN 00502.300 Digest of state guardianship laws*. https://secure.ssa.gov/poms.nsf/lnx/0200502300 (accessed January 23, 2016).

VA (U.S. Department of Veterans Affairs). 2015a. Evaluating competency. In *Compensation and pension manual: Part 3*. Washington, DC: VA. http://www.benefits.va.gov/WARMS/docs/admin21/m21_1/mr/part3/subptiv/ch08/M21-1III_iv_8_SecA.docx (accessed December 15, 2015).

VA. 2015b. General information on the rating activity. In *Compensation and pension manual: Part 3*. Washington, DC: VA. http://www.benefits.va.gov/WARMS/docs/admin21/m21_1/mr/part3/subptiv/ch01/M21-1_III_iv_1.doc (accessed December 15, 2015).

VA. 2015c. Processing awards to incompetent beneficiaries. In *Compensation and pension manual: Part 3*. Washington, DC: VA. http://www.benefits.va.gov/WARMS/docs/admin21/m21_1/mr/part3/subptv/ch09/M21-1III_v_9_SecB.docx (accessed December 15, 2015).

ANNEX TABLE 2-1 Comparison of Social Security Administration and Similar Programs

	Social Security Administration	U.S. Department of Veterans Affairs	Office of Personnel Management	Service Canada
Overall Size	68 million beneficiaries Old Age, Survivor and Disability Insurance (OASDI): 59 million Supplemental Security Income (SSI): 8.3 million	4.25 million beneficiaries Disability: 3.95 million Pension: 300,000	2.5 million annuitants and survivor annuitants	N/A
Beneficiaries with Representative Payee	8.7 million OASDI: 5.6 million SSI: 3.2 million	177,000	16,000	N/A
Presumption of Capability	Yes	Yes	Yes	Yes
Potential Triggers for Questioning Capability	Beneficiary has difficulty • answering questions • getting evidence or information necessary to pursue the claim • understanding explanations and reporting instructions Beneficiary has mental or physical impairment resulting in • severe disorientation • severe impairment of intellect • gross deficit in judgment • inability to communicate	100 percent disability rating for a mental condition Finding of legal incompetence by a court	Correspondence from someone familiar with beneficiary suggesting inability to manage affairs Information received in response to surveys of annuitants Information arising from further inquiry into nonresponse to survey, or survey returned as undeliverable Computerized matching with other benefit programs	Contact from person familiar with beneficiary, such as a family member, friend, or neighbor

continued

ANNEX TABLE 2-1 Continued

	Social Security Administration	U.S. Department of Veterans Affairs	Office of Personnel Management	Service Canada
Types of Evidence Considered	Legal (follows court order when beneficiaries declared legally incompetent) Medical Lay (required if no legal finding of incompetence)	Legal (considered as evidence but nonbinding) Medical (required) Lay	Legal (follows court order when guardian, conservator, or fiduciary appointed for beneficiary by court) Medical (requires statement from treating physician) Lay (requires two affidavits from persons familiar with beneficiary)	Legal (legal arrangements, such as an enduring power of attorney, public trustee, court-appointed committee or guardian, are binding) Combination of medical and lay (Certificate of Incapability form must be filled out by a medical professional—other professional permitted in rare circumstances; queries for information on medical diagnosis, as well as on financial competence and performance)

Appeals Process	Appeals can be made within 60 days Appeals through informal *protest* or formal (in writing) *request for reconsideration* Review of new and existing evidence by claims representative not involved in original decision; face-to-face interview may be requested to resolve any problems If initial determination is upheld, beneficiary may request appeal before an administrative law judge	Appeals, in writing, can be made within 60 days Rating Veterans Service Representative (RVSR) at ratings office collocated with fiduciary hub conducts requested hearings, reviews original and additional evidence, and renders final decision	Appeals can be made within 10 days of decision Beneficiaries may provide additional evidence for review by contract doctor	No formal appeals process for individuals who are deemed incapable, as "any decision by the Department regarding an appointment of a trustee for the purposes of administering CPP [Canada Pension Plan] and/or OAS [Old Age Security] benefits is made under the Minister's discretion and is therefore not appealable"

continued

ANNEX TABLE 2-1 Continued

	Social Security Administration	U.S. Department of Veterans Affairs	Office of Personnel Management	Service Canada
Review	No formal process for ongoing review May be reevaluated whenever there is indication or evidence that incapable beneficiary has become capable or capable beneficiary has become incapable Staff must "consider reviewing"[a] capability in specific situations: • continuing disability reviews • SSI redeterminations • discovery that a beneficiary manages any other benefits • beneficiary appeal • any other contact with the beneficiary or payee that raises a question of capability	The VA field examiners contact incompetent beneficiaries every 1 to 3 years to review both their incompetence ratings and their fiduciaries' performance Competency may also be reviewed any time new medical evidence is received; may include evidence from • hospital summary • report of release to or discharge from nonbed care • report of other material change in condition Upon receipt of evidence, Veterans Service Representative (VSR) refers claims folder for RVSR review	Not specifically for reevaluation of competency Representative payee survey administered every 2 years to ensure benefits expended in best interest of beneficiary; unclear whether information from this survey may trigger reevaluation of competency	Upon initial appointment of trustee, staff "must establish whether the case should be reviewed at a later date in order to determine if the condition of the beneficiary has improved to the extent that the trusteeship should be terminated"[b] When beneficiary informs department that he or she has regained capability When trustee notifies department beneficiary has regained capacity

Instructions to Informants	No formal instructions Suggested questions provided to field office staff for collecting lay evidence, but not provided to informants	No formal instructions	Provides Information Necessary for a Competency Determination (see Appendix C) to physicians and persons providing lay evidence	Provides Certificate of Incapability (see Appendix C)
Unique Aspects and Features		Supervised direct pay	Uses computerized matching with other benefits-paying organizations, including SSA and the U.S. Department of Labor, to analyze benefit disbursement to federal employees that may impact OPM benefits; may provide information that brings capability into question	

[a] "'Consider reviewing' doesn't necessarily mean conducting a full capability development. It means examining the indicators in a case and deciding whether full development is needed" (SSA, 2015c).
[b] SOURCE: Service Canada, 2015b, p. 20.

3

Effects of Appointment of Representative Payees on Beneficiaries

As discussed in the preceding chapters, impairment of the ability to manage or direct the management of one's benefits can lead to the appointment of a third party—in the U.S. Social Security Administration's (SSA's) terminology, a representative payee—to perform that function. Representative payees who appropriately discharge their role can enable beneficiaries who lack financial capability to meet their basic needs and to sustain the quality of their lives. However, empowering another person with control over disbursement of an individual's financial resources also creates risks for improper use or mismanagement of those funds or actual financial abuse. A representative payee's failure to disburse funds appropriately can have life-altering consequences, including insufficient funds to pay for housing, food, and clothing. When an individual lacks these necessities, consequences can include the development or exacerbation of health problems, which may require hospitalization; a decision to turn to criminal activity to obtain money, resulting in legal charges and possible incarceration; and inability to pay rent, which can lead to homelessness or institutionalization (Conrad et al., 2006; Moberg and Rick, 2008). Given the range of potential consequences of the appointment of a representative payee, the committee was asked to consider the effects of SSA's decision to appoint a representative payee on the beneficiary.

BENEFITS ASSOCIATED WITH THE APPOINTMENT OF A REPRESENTATIVE PAYEE

Representative payee programs have been found to have significant positive effects on a beneficiary's ability to live independently, which in turn affects the individual's health and well-being. Appointment of a representative payee is associated with increased ability to meet basic needs (Luchins et al., 2003); declines in homelessness, victimization, and arrests (Rosenheck et al., 1997; Stoner, 1989); and increased adherence to outpatient substance abuse treatment (Ries and Comtois, 1997). For individuals diagnosed with a mental impairment, better money management is associated with superior quality of life, fewer hospitalizations, improved treatment compliance, and greater self-efficacy (Elbogen et al., 2011; Luchins et al., 2003, 2014).

Research results are mixed as to whether the representative payee arrangement reduces substance abuse (Ries et al., 2004) or has no effect (Rosen, 2011; Rosen et al., 2007; Swartz et al., 2003). Even if substance abuse does not decrease, however, clients with representative payees are more likely to stay engaged in substance abuse and mental health treatment (Conrad et al., 2006; Ries and Comtois, 1997). In addition, coordination of a community-based representative payee program with psychiatric and clinical care has been associated with reduced substance use and improved quality of life and money management (Conrad et al., 2006).

In addition to effects on individual beneficiaries, the representative payee program may have positive economic implications for the communities in which beneficiaries live. For beneficiaries with mental illness and/or substance abuse currently involved in community human service programs, these programs provide the oversight needed to maintain household independence, avoid the use of shelters and confinement, and encourage participation in substance abuse treatment. Without independent housing, people often turn to family or friends, or become homeless. The societal cost of homelessness is surprisingly high because of the associated costs of hospitalization, medical treatment, incarceration, police intervention, and emergency shelter expenses (Pinellas County Board of County Commissioners, 2012, p. 22). For example, the average cost to incarcerate an inmate for a year in a community corrections center is $26,163, which is approximately $72 per day (*Federal Register*, 2013). Estimates of the annual cost of chronic homelessness range from $35,000 to $150,000 per person, which is $96 to $411 per day (Henwood et al., 2015). Such expenses often are borne by taxpayers through their local governments.

In sum, the committee recognizes that appointment of a representative payee can have significant positive effects on individual beneficiaries, with notable improvements in their abilities to live independently, and on communities, which can avoid the costs associated with providing institutional care—whether in shelters, residential treatment facilities or correctional facilities—to incapable beneficiaries. However, in addition to such positive effects, appointment of a representative payee also has potential negative consequences.

RISKS ASSOCIATED WITH THE APPOINTMENT OF A REPRESENTATIVE PAYEE

There are potential psychological consequences of having a representative payee appointed to manage one's benefits. Having access to one's money and being able to manage it oneself is, for many people, critical to feelings of self-worth. Being able to control how one's money is spent is considered one of the essential elements of liberty and of self-determination. Loss of control over finances can provoke fear and anxiety, be seen as a threat to autonomy, and encourage dependence (Dixon et al., 1999; Luchins et al., 2014), and having a representative payee may be perceived by the beneficiary as stigmatizing (Elbogen et al., 2008).

A representative payee is most often a friend or family member of the beneficiary, although other individuals (e.g., lawyers) or organizations (e.g., religious or community organizations, mental health centers, nursing or group homes) also may serve in this role. As work on guardianship has demonstrated, the outcome for the person with a guardian is affected by the characteristics of the guardian (Quinn, 2005; Quinn and Krooks, 2012). If the guardian is responsible, committed to keeping the person housed and in the community, and steadfast in allowing maximum personal freedom, the quality of the person's life and the scope of permitted actions may be better than would be the case if the beneficiary were left without such support. If the guardian is not dedicated to the person's best interests, however, having a guardian may reduce the quality of the person's life.

Representative payee arrangements have the potential to significantly impact the beneficiary's relationships with family members or friends serving in this role. Beneficiaries can be negatively affected by strain in their familial relationships resulting from conflict over the money management responsibilities of family members acting as representative payees. Indeed, having a family member who serves as their representative payee or on whom they are otherwise financially dependent has been found to be associated with a significantly increased risk of interpersonal conflict, aggression, and family violence perpetrated by individuals with severe mental illness (Elbogen et al., 2005b, 2008; Estroff et al., 1994, 1998). In one study, the risk of family violence by beneficiaries with severe mental illness doubled when a family member served as representative payee (Elbogen et al., 2008).

Assignment of a representative payee also has potential legal implications. As discussed in greater detail below, assignment of a representative payee infringes on an individual's autonomy and may limit his or her civil liberties. The committee heard about a specific example of the potential legal implications at its first meeting, when SSA described its reporting requirements under the Brady Handgun Violence Prevention Act (Brady

Act).[1] Under the act, any person who "has been adjudicated as a mental defective" is prohibited from possessing a firearm. Such individuals are to be reported to the National Instant Criminal Background Check System (NICS), which gun dealers must check before selling a firearm. Currently, the U.S. Department of Veterans Affairs (VA) reports to the NICS the names of beneficiaries deemed incompetent under its system. At the committee's first meeting (Stanton, 2015) and in further correspondence,[2] SSA reported that it was determining how it must comply with such reporting obligations with regard to beneficiaries deemed incapable. On January 4, 2016, the White House announced that SSA will begin the rulemaking process for reporting to the NICS.

USE OF BENEFITS AS LEVERAGE

Research has shown that, although they are not intended to take on this role, representative payees often attempt to improve treatment adherence, discourage substance use, or encourage other behaviors by using access to benefits as leverage (Appelbaum and Redlich, 2006; Elbogen et al., 2005a). Approximately 30-59 percent of patients report experiencing some form of leveraging (i.e., of access to money or housing, or avoidance of commitment to an institution or incarceration), associated primarily with efforts to reduce substance abuse and frequent hospitalizations (Appelbaum and Redlich, 2006; Elbogen et al., 2003a; Monahan et al., 2001). Attempts to influence a beneficiary's behavior may be carried out in various ways. For example, a community mental health center may disburse benefits only when a treatment group is scheduled, thereby encouraging the beneficiary's attendance. State-wide surveys of mental health center representative payee programs in Illinois and Washington State found disbursement of benefits to be at least moderately linked to avoidance of substance abuse in most programs and tightly linked in a substantial minority of programs. For most programs, receipt of benefits was tied less commonly to engagement in mental health treatment (Hanrahan et al., 2002; Ries and Dyck, 1997).

Leverage, however, can move beyond encouragement of desired behaviors to coercion, with the line between the two not always clear. Indeed, the same behavior may be viewed as leverage by its proponents and as coercion by its critics. Whereas leverage implies an effort to influence the beneficiary's behavior in ways that are believed to be helpful to the person (e.g., avoidance of substance abuse), control of a person's benefits can also be used to compel behaviors for the benefit of the representative payee

---

[1] 18 USC 922.

[2] Personal communication, M. Rochowiak, Office of Disability Policy, SSA, September 21, 2015.

(e.g., demanding performance of work around the house in exchange for access to benefits), in effect exploiting the beneficiary. Beyond coercion, there is also the potential for overt misuse of benefits. For example, representative payees may pay bills with beneficiaries' funds that benefit both the beneficiaries and the payees, such as their rent or food bills, or divert benefits directly for their own purposes. Although an examination of misuse of benefits by a representative payee is beyond the scope of this study, the potential effects of such actions on beneficiaries need to be acknowledged.

Even though leverage may produce several positive outcomes as compared with no use of leverage—for example, less alcohol and drug use and better money management (Ries et al., 2004)—the question of its legitimacy is legally and morally complex. One might argue that leveraging a beneficiary's funds to ensure adherence is in the best interest of the beneficiary. Alternatively, critics might view such action as a violation of the beneficiary's civil liberties (see the discussion of this issue below). To be most effective, leverage must be used carefully. One study found, for example, that clients were more likely to agree that leveraging funds was helpful if they also had opportunities to make decisions regarding their mental health treatment (Elbogen et al., 2005a). (Beneficiaries' perspectives on leveraging of their benefits are discussed further below.) The knowledge base on the effectiveness and consequences of leverage would be expanded by additional research with control groups and alternative treatments, as well as longitudinal studies.

THE BENEFICIARY'S PERSPECTIVE

As discussed above, research has demonstrated many potential benefits and raised some concerns about the impact on the beneficiary of having a representative payee appointed. However, much of this research is based on reports from caregivers, practitioners, and representative payees, and less research has examined the impact from the perspective of the beneficiary. Those studies that have looked at the beneficiary's perspective have explored satisfaction with having a representative payee, views on coercion, and use of funds.

Dixon and colleagues (1999) interviewed 54 clients with persistent mental illness who participated in an inner-city assertive treatment program and their case managers who served as representative payees regarding the benefits and problems associated with having a representative payee. They found that clients' satisfaction with having a case manager as a representative payee was initially low, but the longer clients had a case manager serve as a representative payee, the more satisfied they became. Overall, both clients and case managers reported benefits of having a representative payee in the areas of housing, budgeting, and control of drug and alcohol use. Fifty-three percent of the clients reported feeling very involved in the development of a monthly budget, and only 20 percent reported feeling that having the case manager as the representative payee interfered with the therapeutic process.

Elbogen and colleagues (2005a) explored beneficiaries' feelings about the use of disability funds by representative payees as a way to improve treatment adherence. In this study, 104 clients recently diagnosed with schizophrenia or a related condition were interviewed. A majority (65 percent) of respondents reported that attempts to increase treatment adherence by withholding benefits were unhelpful. Those who felt respected by the representative payee were less likely to see this practice as coercive. Those with higher levels of education were more likely to perceive this strategy as coercive. Additionally, respondents who reported abusing substances in the previous month were less likely to endorse the use of benefits to increase adherence.

Angell and colleagues (2007) explored the effects of having a payee and the experience of "perceived financial leverage"[3] on client–provider relationships. Their sample included 205 adults with mental illness who were receiving services from an urban community mental health clinic. Of those clients with a clinician as a payee, 40 percent reported perceived financial leverage. Clients with a clinician as a payee also reported experiencing more conflict, negativity, and intrusion in the client–practitioner relationship. Based on their analyses, the authors posited that "payeeship leads to strain in the therapeutic relationship when it is used as a mechanism for promoting adherence" (p. 370). Lastly, Elbogen and colleagues (2003b) conducted a study of persons hospitalized with a diagnosis of a psychotic or major affective disorder. A minority of clients with representative payees reported insufficient money to cover basic expenses such as housing, food, and shelter. However, 43 percent reported not having enough spending money for enjoyable activities. This complaint was more common among those whose representative payee was not a family member. As the authors note, lack of spending money may be highly problematic given the importance of social skills and social networks for individuals with severe mental disorders.

Taken together, this literature suggests that while beneficiaries may perceive some benefits to having a representative payee, such as maintaining stable housing, those who have a clinician as representative payee may perceive this arrangement as coercive and may experience a loss of

[3] Respondents were categorized as experiencing perceived financial leverage based on an affirmative response to questions regarding (1) "whether the payee had ever withheld money until the respondent followed through on mental health treatment, alcohol or drug treatment, or taking medication"; or (2) "whether, in the past six months, anyone had made them feel as though they would not receive spending money if they did not attend treatment appointments or take medications" (Angell et al., 2007, pp. 366-367).

autonomy. However, the literature in this area is sparse and includes only individuals with mental illness, leaving the perspectives of other beneficiaries unexplored.

MINIMIZING THE IMPACT ON AUTONOMY OF HAVING A REPRESENTATIVE PAYEE

As noted above, appointing a representative payee raises legal issues related to individual civil liberties; it also raises philosophical issues of autonomy, societal responsibility, and justified paternalism. On the one hand, individuals who have reached adulthood are presumed to possess moral agency and legal rights that, in general, protect their decisions about personal health and well-being, how they spend their money, and how they manage their affairs. On the other hand, clear observation and a review of the available data on incapacity demonstrate that in many adults, the ability to exercise their moral agency and legal rights is restricted by developmental delay, neurodegenerative disorders, mental illness, or physical impairment. To deem someone incapable when he or she is not erodes personal liberty, creates stigma through labeling, deprives the person of the freedom to direct personally appropriate actions based on long-held values and preferences, and creates opportunities for exploitation. Alternatively, to permit someone incapable of clear inner direction to continue to manage his or her personal financial affairs may cause the person preventable harm resulting from mismanagement of funds and an increased potential for victimization by others.

Ultimately, the decision to appoint a representative payee entails weighing the beneficiary's personal autonomy and preferences, or what remains after impairment, against paternalistic intervention meant to protect his or her best interests. *Autonomy* has been defined as "personal rule of the self that is free from both controlling interferences by others and from personal limitations that prevent meaningful choice" (Pantilat, 2008). In the case of persons needing a representative payee, however, it is precisely the personal limitations that demand the help of others. In such cases, a paternalistic approach may be warranted. For the purposes of this discussion, *paternalism* is defined as "the interference of a state or an individual with another person, against their will, and defended or motivated by a claim that the person interfered with will be better off or protected from harm. . . . At the theoretical level it raises questions of how persons should be treated when they are less than fully rational" (Dworkin, 2014). Such paternalism is commonly evident in a variety of contexts, such as legal (e.g., seatbelt laws, motorcycle helmet laws, antidrug legislation), medical (e.g., a physician withholding information about a patient's condition), and medico-legal (e.g., civil commitment, requiring minors to have blood transfusions despite religious prohibition). In the case of SSA representative payment, the role of the payee is to ensure that the person is sheltered and has sufficient money for food, shelter, and clothing, thus being protected from the consequences of his or her impairments and not becoming a burden on family and society.

SUPPORTED DECISION MAKING

It is also important to recognize that the decision to appoint a representative payee need not vitiate autonomy and substitute strict paternalism. Over the past few decades, the field of medicine increasingly has moved away from a paternalistic approach, with clinicians making decisions on behalf of patients according to their perceptions of patients' best interests, toward a concept of shared decision making. *Shared decision making* in medicine has been defined as

> a model of patient-centered care that enables and encourages people to play a role in the management of their own health. It operates under the premise that, armed with good information, consumers can and will participate in the medical decision-making process by asking informed questions and expressing personal values and opinions about their conditions and treatment options. (AHRQ, n.d.)

Such a model brings together the clinician's expertise and the patient's preferences, values, and opinions to reach a decision on important health care choices. Research has shown that the benefits of this model include increased patient satisfaction, more favorable health outcomes, and lower demand for health care resources (AHRQ, n.d.).

In a similar fashion, society has become increasingly attuned to assisting persons with disabilities in maximizing their intellectual potential and enhancing their moral authority with respect to decisions about their lives. Accordingly, recent years have seen a call by disability rights activists to move away from the traditional model of *surrogate decision making*, in which individuals are authorized to make decisions for persons with intellectual and cognitive disabilities, to a model of *supported decision making*, which acknowledges that some elements of autonomy—of holding values and preferences—survive despite these disabilities and are deserving of support by others.

Such a model has increasingly been encouraged or endorsed both in the United States and internationally. For example, courts in New York[4] and Virginia[5,6] have ruled in favor of persons with intellectual disabilities

---

[4] In Re: the Guardianship of Dameris L., Pursuant to SCPA Article 17-A.

[5] *Ross et al. v. Hatch*, 2013.

[6] See http://supporteddecisionmaking.org/sites/default/files/ross_hatch_trial_court_decision.pdf (accessed February 23, 2016).

seeking to terminate guardianship in favor of a supported decision-making model that assists and supports autonomy instead of superseding it. In 2015, Texas enacted Senate Bill 1881, enabling an adult with a disability to "voluntarily, without undue influence or coercion, enter into a supported decision-making agreement with a supporter."[7] The U.S. Department of Health and Human Services' Administration for Community Living has endorsed this model as well, and provided funding for the creation of a national training, technical assistance, and resource center (the National Resource Center for Supported Decision Making) to gather and disseminate data and generate research on shared decision making (Bishop and Walker, 2015). The VA, as discussed in Chapter 2, uses a similar model (supervised direct payment) in certain cases in which a beneficiary is rated incompetent but determined to be capable of managing his or her benefits with supervision. Internationally, Article 12 of the United Nations Convention on the Rights of Persons with Disabilities recognizes that "persons with disabilities enjoy legal capacity on an equal basis with others," including the right to manage their financial affairs, and should be provided, when needed, the support necessary to exercise their legal capacity.[8] Many countries, including Australia, Canada, and Sweden, among others, have increasingly supported such a model.

The concept of supported decision making can inform perspectives on determining a beneficiary's need for a representative payee. With proper support, some beneficiaries who might otherwise require the appointment of a representative payee may be able to manage or direct the management of their benefits. For example, beneficiaries with disabilities who are prone to fluctuations in financial capability may be provided support proportional to their needs as situations dictate.

Supported decision making also can inform the role of the representative payee. Representative payees endorsing and using a supported decision-making model may encourage the expression of preferences, beliefs, and values; foster collaboration in decision making; provide skills training to improve financial competence and performance; and ensure opportunities for beneficiaries to make independent decisions, whenever possible. When supported decision making is pursued appropriately, a person with a representative payee may have more actual control over his or her life than someone without such support.

---

[7] See http://www.capitol.state.tx.us/BillLookup/BillSummary.aspx?LegSess=84R&Bill=SB1881 (accessed February 23, 2016).

[8] See http://www.un.org/disabilities/default.asp?id=272 (accessed February 23, 2016).

SUMMARY

This chapter has examined the effects of appointment of a representative payee on the beneficiary, which may include significant health (physical and mental), social, familial, and financial impacts. The consequential nature of appointing a representative payee implies the need to make such decisions with great care and the best evidence available.

Representative payees who appropriately discharge their role can enable beneficiaries who lack financial capability to meet their basic needs and to sustain the quality of their lives. Representative payee programs can have significant positive effects on a beneficiary's ability to live independently; meet basic needs; avoid hospitalization, homelessness, victimization, or arrest; remain engaged in substance abuse treatment; and increase quality of life. Such programs may also have positive economic implications for communities in which beneficiaries live, which can avoid the costs associated with providing institutional care to incapable beneficiaries.

However, appointment of a representative payee also has potential negative effects. Loss of control over finances can have psychological consequences, affecting feelings of self-worth, provoking fear and anxiety, encouraging dependence, and threatening autonomy. Relationships with family members or friends who serve as representative payees can be strained by conflict over money management. Additionally, empowering another person with control over disbursement of an individual's financial resources creates risks for improper use or mismanagement of those funds or actual financial abuse.

Although they are not intended to take on this role, research shows that representative payees may also try to leverage access to benefits to improve treatment adherence, discourage substance use, or encourage other behaviors. Leverage, however, can move beyond encouragement of desired behaviors to coercion, with the line between the two not always being clear. While leverage implies attempts to influence the beneficiary's behavior in ways that are beneficial to the individual, control over an individual's benefits can also be used to compel behaviors for the benefit of the representative payee, in effect exploiting the beneficiary.

Although limited, research on the beneficiary's perspective suggests that beneficiaries have mixed feelings about the appointment of a representative payee, with positive feelings growing over time. Although beneficiaries may perceive some benefits to having a representative payee, such as maintaining stable housing, improved budgeting, and control of drug and alcohol use, beneficiaries who have clinicians as representative payees may view this arrangement as coercive and may perceive a loss of autonomy.

Ultimately, the decision to appoint a representative payee entails weighing the beneficiary's personal autonomy and preferences, or what remains after impairment, against paternalistic intervention meant to protect his or her best interests. However, appointing a representative payee need not vitiate autonomy and substitute strict paternalism. A supported decision-making model can inform perspectives on determining the need for and the role of the representative payee, and provide a foundation for a relationship that positively impacts the beneficiary. Representative payees endorsing and using such a model may encourage the expression of preferences, beliefs, and values; foster collaboration in decision making; and provide opportunities for beneficiaries to make independent decisions, whenever possible. Appropriate use of this model may provide a beneficiary with greater control over his or her life relative to someone without such support.

REFERENCES

AHRQ (Agency for Healthcare Research and Quality). n.d. *Shared decision-making.* https://cahps.ahrq.gov/quality-improvement/improvement-guide/6-strategies-for-improving/communication/Shared-Decision-Making/index.html (accessed January 29, 2016).

Angell, B., N. I. Martinez, C. A. Mahoney, and P. W. Corrigan. 2007. Payeeship, financial leverage, and the client-provider relationship. *Psychiatric Services* 58(3):365-372.

Appelbaum, P. S., and A. Redlich. 2006. Use of leverage over patients' money to promote adherence to psychiatric treatment. *The Journal of Nervous and Mental Disease* 194(4):294-302.

Bishop, A., and E. Walker. 2015. Preserving the right to self-determination: Supported decision-making. *ACL Blog.* http://www.acl.gov/NewsRoom/blog/2015/2015_01_28.aspx (accessed January 29, 2016).

Conrad, K. J., G. Lutz, M. D. Matters, L. Donner, E. Clark, and P. Lynch. 2006. Randomized trial of psychiatric care with representative payeeship for persons with serious mental illness. *Psychiatric Services (Washington, D.C.)* 57(2):197-204.

Dixon, L., J. Turner, N. Krauss, J. Scott, and S. McNary. 1999. Case managers' and clients' perspectives on a representative payee program. *Psychiatric Services (Washington, D.C.)* 50(6):781-786.

Dworkin, G. 2014. Paternalism. *The Stanford Encyclopedia of Philosophy* (Summer 2014 Edition). http://plato.stanford.edu/archives/sum2014/entries/paternalism (accessed January 29, 2016).

Elbogen, E. B., J. W. Swanson, and M. S. Swartz. 2003a. Psychiatric disability, the use of financial leverage, and perceived coercion in mental health services. *International Journal of Forensic Mental Health* 2(2):119-127.

Elbogen, E. B., J. W. Swanson, M. S. Swartz, and H. R. Wagner. 2003b. Characteristics of third-party money management for persons with psychiatric disabilities. *Psychiatric Services* 54(8):1136-1141.

Elbogen, E. B., C. Soriano, R. V. Dorn, M. S. Swartz, and J. W. Swanson. 2005a. Consumer views of representative payee use of disability funds to leverage treatment adherence. *Psychiatric Services (Washington, D.C.)* 56(1):45-49.

Elbogen, E. B., J. W. Swanson, M. S. Swartz, and R. Van Dorn. 2005b. Family representative payeeship and violence risk in severe mental illness. *Law and Human Behavior* 29(5):563-574.

Elbogen, E. B., C. Wilder, M. S. Swartz, and J. W. Swanson. 2008. Caregivers as money managers for adults with severe mental illness: How treatment providers can help. *Academic Psychiatry* 32(2):104-110.

Elbogen, E. B., J. Tiegreen, C. Vaughan, and D. W. Bradford. 2011. Money management, mental health, and psychiatric disability: A recovery-oriented model for improving financial skills. *Psychiatric Rehabilitation Journal* 34(3):223-231.

Estroff, S. E., C. Zimmer, W. S. Lachicotte, and J. Benoit. 1994. The influence of social networks and social support on violence by persons with serious mental illness. *Psychiatric Services* 45(7):669-679.

Estroff, S. E., J. W. Swanson, W. S. Lachicotte, M. Swartz, and M. Bolduc. 1998. Risk reconsidered: Targets of violence in the social networks of people with serious psychiatric disorders. *Social Psychiatry and Psychiatric Epidemiology* 33(1):S95-S101.

Federal Register. 2013. *Annual determination of average cost of incarceration*. Washington, DC: Office of the General Counsel, Federal Bureau of Prisons. https://www.federalregister.gov/articles/2013/03/18/2013-06139/annual-determination-of-average-cost-of-incarceration (accessed January 29, 2016).

Hanrahan, P., D. J. Luchins, C. Savage, G. Patrick, D. Roberts, and K. J. Conrad. 2002. Representative payee programs for persons with mental illness in Illinois. *Psychiatric Services (Washington, D.C.)* 53(2):190-194.

Henwood, B. F., S. L. Wenzel, P. F. Mangano, M. Hombs, D K. Padgett, T. Byrne, E. Rice, S. C. Butts, and M. C. Uretsky. 2015. *The grand challenge of ending homelessness* (Grand Challenges for Social Work Initiative Working Paper No. 10). Cleveland, OH: American Academy of Social Work and Social Welfare.

Luchins, D., D. Roberts, and P. Hanrahan. 2003. Representative payeeship and mental illness: A review. *Administration in Policy in Mental Health* 30(4):341-353.

Luchins, D. J., P. Hanrahan, K. J. Conrad, C. Savage, M. D. Matters, and M. Shinderman. 2014. An agency-based representative payee program and improved community tenure of persons with mental illness. *Psychiatric Services (Washington, D.C.)* 49(9):1218-1222.

Moberg, P. J., and J. H. Rick. 2008. Decision-making capacity and competency in the elderly: A clinical and neuropsychological perspective. *NeuroRehabilitation* 23(5):403-413.

Monahan, J., R. J. Bonnie, P. S. Appelbaum, P. S. Hyde, H. J. Steadman, and M. S. Swartz. 2001. Mandated community treatment: Beyond outpatient commitment. *Psychiatric Services (Washington, D.C.)* 52(9):1198-1205.

Pantilat, S. 2008. *Autonomy vs. beneficence*. http://missinglink.ucsf.edu/lm/ethics/Content%20Pages/fast_fact_auton_bene.htm (accessed February 9, 2016).

Pinellas County Board of County Commissioners. 2012. *Workshop session: The economic impact of poverty*. http://www.stpete.org/oldsite/economic_development_dept/redevelopment_initiatives/docs/PSSCRA/May_2012___Pinellas_County___Economic_Impact_of_Poverty.pdf (accessed February 11, 2016).

Quinn, M. J. 2005. *Guardianship of adults: Achieving justice, autonomy, and safety*. New York: Springer.

Quinn, M. J., and H. S. Crooks. 2012. The relationship between the guardian and the court. *Utah Law Review* 2012(3):1611-1666.

Ries, R. K., and K. A. Comtois. 1997. Managing disability benefits as part of treatment for persons with severe mental illness and comorbid drug/alcohol disorders: A comparative study of payee and non-payee participants. *American Journal on Addictions* 6(4):330-338.

Ries, R. K., and D. G. Dyck. 1997. Representative payee practices of community mental health centers in Washington State. *Psychiatric Services (Washington, D.C.)* 48(6):811-814.

Ries, R. K., D. G. Dyck, R. Short, D. Srebnik, A. Fisher, and K. A. Comtois. 2004. Outcomes of managing disability benefits among patients with substance dependence and severe mental illness. *Psychiatric Services (Washington, D.C.)* 55(4):445-447.

Rosen, M. I. 2011. The "check effect" reconsidered. *Addiction* 106(6):1071-1077.

Rosen, M. I., T. J. McMahon, and R. Rosenheck. 2007. Does assigning a representative payee reduce substance abuse? *Drug and Alcohol Dependence* 86(2):115-122.

Rosenheck, R., J. Lam, and F. Randolph. 1997. Impact of representative payees on substance use by homeless persons with serious mental illness. *Psychiatric Services (Washington, D.C.)* 48(6):800-806.

Stanton, S. 2015. Opening remarks and overview of the SSA capability determination process. Presentation to the Committee to Evaluate the Social Security Administration's Capability Determination Process for Adult Beneficiaries, February 3, Washington, DC.

Stoner, M. R. 1989. Money management services for the homeless mentally ill. *Hospital and Community Psychiatry* 40(7):751-763.

Swartz, J. A., C. M. Hsieh, and J. Baumohl. 2003. Disability payments, drug use and representative payees: An analysis of the relationships. *Addiction* 98(7):965-975.

4

Abilities Required to Manage and Direct the Management of Benefits

As discussed in Chapter 2, the U.S. Social Security Administration (SSA) uses the term *capability* to refer to "a beneficiary's ability to manage or direct the management of his [or] her Social Security funds" (SSA, 2015b). *Incapability* is a determination by SSA that an individual beneficiary is unable to manage or direct the management of his or her benefits as a result of mental disability or, sometimes, physical disability. Akin to the legal definition of *incompetence*,[1] incapability is a dichotomous determination made by an authoritative body. Making such a determination requires an assessment of the individual's *financial capability*.

For SSA to consider an individual capable, he or she must be able either to *manage* or to *direct the management* of his or her benefits. Although the abilities required to manage and to direct the management of one's funds clearly overlap, there are differences as well. *Managing* one's own funds means one is fully and independently responsible for managing the funds in a way that routinely meets one's needs and goals. If one can manage one's funds, one presumably also can direct the management of the funds. Even if someone is not capable of fully and independently managing his or her own funds, that person may still be capable of *directing the management* of the funds by someone else. For example, people with a mental impairment may be able to direct another to manage their funds based on their goals, such as

[1] In legal terms, *incompetency* refers to a determination by the courts that an individual is unable to manage his or her affairs as a result of mental disability or, sometimes, physical disability. SSA uses the term "legally incompetent" to refer to one subset of beneficiaries who will automatically receive a representative payee.

paying rent on time so as not to lose their apartment, even though they themselves are not able to perform the day-to-day tasks necessary to achieve those goals. Similarly, people who are mentally capable of managing their own funds but have a physical impairment, such as quadriplegia or an inability to speak, that makes them physically unable to accomplish the tasks required may still be able to direct someone else to perform those tasks for them.

As discussed in Chapter 1, the committee broadens SSA's conception of *capability* to encompass the full realm of one's finances, defining the term *financial capability* as managing or directing the management of one's funds in a way that routinely meets one's needs and goals. In the context of SSA, *financial capability* refers to a beneficiary's managing or directing the management of SSA funds in a way that routinely[2] meets his or her basic needs. *Financial competence* and *financial performance* both contribute to financial capability (see Figure 1-1 in Chapter 1). This chapter provides a conceptual overview of these components of financial capability and the cognitive and behavioral processes underlying them. It also includes discussion of mental and physical disorders that may affect financial capability. Chapter 5 addresses methods and measures for assessing financial capability.

FINANCIAL COMPETENCE

Financial competence refers to the financial skills one possesses, as demonstrated through *financial knowledge* and *financial judgment*, typically assessed in a controlled (e.g., office or clinical) setting. *Financial performance* refers to one's degree of success in handling financial demands in the context of the stresses, supports, contextual cues, and resources in one's actual environment (i.e., the actual use of one's financial knowledge and judgment in concrete, real-life situations). For example, a person may be fully competent in appreciating the importance of retirement savings, but at the level of performance may not have sufficient self-control, foresight, or planning skills to actually save money for retirement. Individuals must both decide on their financial goals and take the steps necessary to influence the realization of those goals to possess successful financial self-management. Thus, successful financial performance involves intact cognitive and behavioral components. Importantly, these are complex interactions that cannot be reduced to a single score or algorithm. As Lichtenberg (2015) notes, "People are more than the sum of their cognitive abilities."

[2] The committee recognizes that circumstances and personal preferences at times may require or lead individuals to forgo a basic need, such as food. Nevertheless, individuals' overall behavior may still reflect an ability to use their benefits to meet their basic needs over time. When that occurs, their needs are being met routinely, in the sense in which that term is used in this report.

Financial Knowledge

The first component of financial competence is *financial knowledge*, which encompasses the declarative and procedural knowledge required for the effective management of one's finances. *Declarative knowledge* refers to knowing that something is the case. As it relates to financial knowledge, declarative knowledge is "the ability to describe facts, concepts, and events related to financial activities" (Marson, 2015; Marson et al., 2000; Moye and Marson, 2007, p. P7), such as arithmetic knowledge (e.g., basic numeracy), semantic and conceptual knowledge of financial terms and associated concepts (e.g., currency values, bills, checks), and knowledge of one's finances (e.g., how much money one has). Requirements for declarative financial knowledge are evolving with technological advances. For example, successful financial management today may involve the use of ATMs (automated teller machines) and online banking. In some cases (e.g., severe intellectual disability), individuals may never acquire sufficient declarative financial knowledge to be able to manage or direct the management of their finances. In other cases (e.g., neurodegenerative processes such as Alzheimer's disease or semantic dementia), individuals may lose their semantic and conceptual knowledge of financial terms and concepts (e.g., paying bills, using currency) and other aspects of financial knowledge, including knowledge of their assets, income, and the like.

Procedural knowledge refers to knowing how to do something. Procedural financial knowledge is "the ability to carry out motor based, overlearned practical financial skills and routines such as making change and writing checks," as well as online banking procedures (Marson, 2015; Marson et al., 2000; Moye and Marson, 2007, p. P7). An individual may possess or retain some level of declarative financial knowledge yet lack or have lost the procedural knowledge required to execute the appropriate behavior. For example, a woman with "more advanced" dementia "was observed to grapple with calculating what payment a cleaner required and how to count the necessary money, nonetheless, she was readily able to identify that he was doing a routine job for the couple and therefore needed to be paid" (Boyle, 2013, p. 559). Such individuals still may be able to direct the management of their financial affairs even though they have lost the procedural knowledge required to perform the actions themselves. On the other hand, a study of individuals with mild cognitive impairment indicated that they retained the purely procedural task of cash transactions, while other performance skills (e.g., bill payment, understanding and using a bank statement) with more complex conceptual components were compromised (Okonkwo et al., 2006).

Financial knowledge is cognitively mediated and influenced by contextual factors related to the environment and the person. *Environmental factors* include individuals' opportunities to acquire the declarative and procedural knowledge required for financial competence. *Personal factors* include the presence of psychiatric (e.g., schizophrenia, bipolar disorder), neurologic (e.g., traumatic brain injury, dementia, mild cognitive impairment, stroke), and other medical (e.g., disorders associated with severe pain, debilitation, or hypoxia) conditions (Marson, 2013) that may affect individuals' cognitive function. It is worth noting that financial knowledge encompasses a wide range of declarative and procedural knowledge—from basic financial transactions (purchases, bill paying) to investing and compound interest. For SSA's purposes of determining financial capability, the committee is concerned primarily with the basic knowledge and skills individuals must have to use their benefits to meet their basic needs for food, shelter, and clothing.

Financial Judgment

The second component of financial competence is *financial judgment*, defined by the committee as possession of the abilities required to make financial decisions and choices that serve the individual's best interests.[3] As discussed in Chapter 1, the committee recognizes the subjective nature of determining an individual's "best interests" and has adopted the minimally restrictive standard of satisfying the basic needs of food, shelter, and clothing for purposes of this report. The committee understands that personal values will affect the ways in which individuals choose to satisfy their basic needs. In addition, when financial resources are limited, individuals often must decide which of their basic needs will take priority, and personal values will affect those decisions as well.

Decision making in the financial realm, like decision making for medical treatment or for participation in research, can be viewed as a specific area of decision making more broadly. The abilities required to make financial decisions and choices in one's best interests (financial judgment) can be extrapolated from the extensive literature on decision-making capacity in medical and research contexts. Various authors have postulated requisite components of decision-making capacity for the purpose of consenting to medical treatment (Appelbaum and Grisso, 1988; Drane, 1985; President's Commission for the Study of Ethical Problems in Medicine and Biomedical and Behavioral Research, 1982; Roth et al., 1977; Tepper and Elwork, 1984). During the past 30 years, consensus has formed around

---

[3] Marson and colleagues (2000) identify judgment as the third component, along with declarative and procedural knowledge, of what they call financial capacity. They define judgment as "the ability to make financial decisions consistent with self-interest, in both everyday and also novel or ambiguous situations" (Moye and Marson, 2007, p. P7).

four abilities that are relevant to individuals' capacity to make treatment decisions (Grisso, 2005, pp. 398-399; see also Charland, 2015; Moye and Marson, 2007)[4]:

- The ability to communicate a choice refers both to the ability to indicate a choice among a variety of alternatives and to "the ability to maintain and communicate stable choices long enough for them to be implemented" (Appelbaum and Grisso, 1988, p. 1635). This does not mean that a person's choices may not vary over time, only that repeated, rapid reversals of choice without reasonable justification may indicate impaired decision making. Impaired consciousness, thought disorders, impaired short-term memory, or an extreme degree of ambivalence may disrupt an individual's ability to communicate reasonably consistent choices (Appelbaum and Grisso, 1988).
- The ability to understand relevant information includes an individual's abilities to receive and remember information relevant to the decision and to comprehend that information, as well as to understand causal relations, associated risks and benefits, the likelihood of different outcomes, and the individual's role in the decision-making process (Appelbaum and Grisso, 1988). These abilities may be impaired by deficits in attention, intelligence, and memory.
- The ability to appreciate the relevance of the information extends the notion of a person's comprehension of relevant information to an appreciation of what that information means for the individual in his or her particular situation. The person recognizes how the information applies to and is significant for his or her own circumstances. Such appreciation includes the values that the individual places on each risk and benefit or potential outcome. The ability to appreciate the relevance of information may be impaired by pathologic distortions or denials stemming from cognitive or affective impairment or a delusional perception of the nature of one's situation (Appelbaum and Grisso, 1988).
- The ability to manipulate information rationally refers to the use of logical processes to compare and weigh the various risks and benefits associated with different courses of action and to reach

[4] Some authors recognize a stable and minimally consistent set of personal values as a fifth element of decision-making capacity (Buchanan and Brock, 1989, pp. 24-25; Charland, 2015; President's Commission for the Study of Ethical Problems in Medicine and Biomedical and Behavioral Research, 1982, pp. 57-58). Personal values play a role in individuals' weighing of risks and benefits and selection among alternative choices (Charland, 1998, 2015; President's Commission for the Study of Ethical Problems in Medicine and Biomedical and Behavioral Research, 1982).

> conclusions that are logically consistent. A number of factors can affect these processes, including "psychotic thought disorder, delirium and dementia, extreme phobia or panic, anxiety, euphoria, depression, and anger" (Appelbaum and Grisso, 1988, p. 1636).

Although studied in the context of medical decision-making capacity, this model is applicable to other decisional contexts, such as financial decision making, as well.

Lichtenberg (2015) highlights the importance of metacognition and self-awareness in decision making and successful financial interactions. Persons with impaired self-awareness may perceive that they are managing their finances effectively but in fact may be making errors and experiencing negative consequences (Hsu and Willis, 2013; Okonkwo et al., 2008; Williamson et al., 2010). Additionally, there is a risk that those with access to money but with limited decision-making capacity may be vulnerable to undue influence and potential fraud. Self-awareness, the ability to evaluate one's performance, and the ability to make adjustments in response to feedback are related to executive functioning. Individuals with developmental or acquired brain injuries, as well as those with dementia or severe psychiatric disorders, are vulnerable to impairment of metacognition. Substance use and dependence can lead to difficulties with working memory, impulsivity, planning, problem solving, and decision making. Importantly, some individuals with conditions such as dementia associated with Parkinson's disease or early frontotemporal dementia may retain basic skills related to financial knowledge but suffer from impaired judgment and the inability to use those skills to meet their needs or protect their interests (Marson, 2013). The cognitive domains relevant to financial competence are reviewed below.

Cognitive Domains Relevant to Financial Competence

The cognitive domains relevant to financial competence (knowledge and judgment) include general cognitive/intellectual ability, attention and vigilance, learning and memory, and executive function (Knight and Marson, 2012; Okonkwo et al., 2006), as well as social cognition and language and communication. These domains should be not viewed as discrete functions but rather as interrelated and overlapping. For example, intact attention is required for an individual to learn and remember information. Thus, although the cognitive domains are discussed separately here, the committee appreciates that the interactions among them are complex, and that noncognitive factors may influence each domain as a whole as well as the "micro-level skills" each entails.

General Cognitive/Intellectual Ability

General cognitive/intellectual ability includes reasoning, problem solving, and meeting cognitive demands of varying complexity (IOM, 2015, p. 146). Intellectual disability affects functioning to varying degrees in three areas: conceptual (e.g., memory, language, reading, writing, math, knowledge acquisition); social (e.g., empathy, social judgment, interpersonal skills, ability to form and to maintain friendships); and practical (e.g., self-management in such areas as money management) (American Psychiatric Association, 2013, p. 37). Impaired cognitive/intellectual ability can affect individuals' acquisition of the math concepts and skills needed for financial competence. Written math skills have been identified as the primary predictor of overall financial competence[5] (Sherod et al., 2009).

Attention and Vigilance

Attention and vigilance are essential components of higher levels of multifactorial cognitive processing and memory. The Occupational Information Development Advisory Panel (OIDAP, 2009) established by SSA defines attention and vigilance as constituting the ability to focus sustained attention in an environment with ordinary distractions. Impairments in this domain may result in difficulties in attending to complex input, holding new information in mind, and performing mental calculations (IOM, 2015, p. 148). Poor or fluctuating attention may make an individual incapable of executing mathematical calculations, paying bills, managing a bank statement, making financial decisions, or conducting financial interactions. Impaired attention is common in individuals with psychosis, depression, dementia, brain injuries, and substance use.

Learning and Memory

Learning and memory refer to the ability to acquire, store, and retrieve information (OIDAP, 2009). New information must be encoded and available to remember and use later. Within the financial context, individuals need to remember account balances, income, expenses over a specified time (i.e., month to month), and procedures for paying bills. Memory impairment can negatively affect financial competence, with serious consequences such as forgetting to pay bills, which may lead to eviction, and the inability to track missing funds from a bank account. Verbal memory has been identified as a secondary predictor of financial competence (Sherod et al., 2009).

---

[5] Although the authors of this study use the term financial capacity, their use of the term, which captures "a range of conceptual, procedural, and judgment skills" (Sherod et al., 2009, p. 259), is similar to the committee's use of *financial competence*.

Another study found the central executive component of working memory, which may be impaired in individuals with histories of substance dependence (Bechara and Martin, 2004), to be strongly correlated with basic monetary skills, checkbook management, bank statement management, and bill payment (Earnst et al., 2001). Learning deficits can impair one's ability to learn the basic skills (e.g., math, manipulating currency) needed to manage finances as well as to acquire new skills, such as how to use an ATM or online banking procedures. Learning and memory deficits are common in those with serious psychiatric disorders, dementia, traumatic brain injuries, and a host of neurologic conditions.

Prospective memory is the process of remembering to perform an action or intention at a future point in time (McDaniel and Einstein, 2000). Prospective memory is directly related to financial competence and performance when an individual must remember to perform a financial task or to make financial decisions that are important to daily living. For example, people may need to remember on the first of the month to pay their rent, utilities, and other bills or transfer money to an account or to conduct some other aspect of financial management. Deficits in prospective memory have been related to declines in financial competence among individuals with Parkinson's disease (Pirogovsky et al., 2012), as well as to decreased functional performance in HIV-seropositive individuals (Woods et al., 2008). Thus, it is reasonable to consider prospective memory a potentially important factor in the ability to carry out one's financial obligations.

Kliegel and colleagues (2002) describe four phases of prospective memory: intention formation, intention retention, intention initiation, and intention execution. Planning, as a part of executive functioning, is critical to forming an intention (e.g., I need to pay rent). In this phase, a person focuses on relevant information while ignoring irrelevant details. An interval then occurs between forming the intention and actually performing the task. During this second phase, intention retention, the individual performs other activities while needing to remember the intention, such as paying his or her rent on time. The amount of time that elapses (e.g., the month between rental payments) and the number of other activities vary. In the third phase, the person must initiate fulfillment of the intention at the defined time (e.g., get cash or a check to pay rent on the first of the month). In this complex phase, several high-level executive functions are involved, including monitoring processes, cognitive flexibility, and inhibition. Additionally, cues (e.g., using a calendar or phone reminder) may prompt the individual to begin to execute the intention. In the fourth phase, the person must fully execute the intention (e.g., deliver the cash or check to the intended payee).

Deficits in prospective memory have been widely observed in mild traumatic brain injury and may be observed in the absence of deficits in retrospective memory (Bisiacchi et al., 1996; Palmer and McDonald,

2000). Increasing evidence also indicates that deficits in prospective memory are observed in individuals with amnestic mild cognitive impairment (Hernandez-Cardenache et al., 2014; Karantzoulis et al., 2009; Kazui et al., 2005).

Executive Function

Executive function is a multidimensional construct that overlaps with aspects of attention and memory, as well as many other cognitive domains. Executive function enables individuals to engage in independent, purposeful behavior. Its components include planning, prioritizing, emotional functioning, organizing, reasoning, problem solving, decision making, responding to feedback and error correction, mental flexibility, overriding impulses, and providing inhibition (American Psychiatric Association, 2013; Elliott, 2003; OIDAP, 2009). Executive function has been identified as a predictor of financial competence (Sherod et al., 2009; see also Earnst et al., 2001; Griffith et al., 2010; Okonkwo et al., 2006). In the context of financial management, it is critical to understanding finances, prioritizing financial obligations, executing multistep behaviors, and directing responsible spending. In financial transactions, individuals need first to understand the concept of paying bills and which bills should be paid. Next, they need to prioritize bills and other financial obligations (e.g., rent, food, clothing, health care). They must then complete multiple steps either to execute online payment or to order and write checks, ensure the deposit of sufficient funds in their bank accounts, buy stamps for mailing, and ultimately mail the bills. Impaired executive function can result in disjointed and disinhibited behavior; impaired judgment, organization, planning, and decision making; and difficulty focusing on more than one task at a time (Elliot, 2003; see also IOM, 2015). In the financial realm, impaired executive function can lead to unnecessary purchases or withdrawals and inability to manage one's financial commitments.

Social Cognition

Social cognition—the cognitive process responsible for helping individuals make sense of other people and themselves (Fiske and Taylor, 2013)—refers to the encoding, storage, retrieval, and processing of information and action planning with respect to other human beings and the world. Social cognition plays a major role in social and emotional development by enabling individuals to take advantage of being part of a social group (Frith and Frith, 2012). One way in which people make sense of social stimuli is by understanding such indicators as facial expressions, body gestures, physical positioning of groups of people, and tone of voice, which signal certain perceptions of fear, disgust, security, contentment, guidance or detection of sought-after goals, and the like. Social cognition can be developed through direct instruction, such as that which occurs between a parent and child during the transfer of knowledge about preferences, attitudes, and reactions concerning objects, people, and situations. The individual learns how to avoid danger, differentiate between good and not-so-good others, and problem solve to attain goals (Fiske and Taylor, 2013; Frith and Frith, 2012).

Impaired social cognition can interfere with one's ability to accurately read social cues that may signal financial schemes, fraudulent activity, identity theft, and the like. Engaging in financial deals or products that "sound too good to be true" may indicate problems with social cognition (among other processes) and contribute to situations in which people with disabilities are susceptible to financial exploitation.

Language and Communication

The domain of language and communication focuses on receptive and expressive language abilities, including the ability to understand spoken or written language, communicate thoughts, and follow directions (American Psychiatric Association, 2013; OIDAP, 2009). In the *International Classification of Functioning, Disability and Health* (*ICF*), the World Health Organization (WHO) distinguishes language from communication, describing the former in terms of mental functioning and the latter in terms of activities (the execution of tasks) and participation (involvement in a life situation) (WHO, 2001) (the *ICF* framework is discussed in greater detail later in this chapter). The mental functions of language include reception of language (i.e., decoding messages to obtain their meaning), expression of language (i.e., production of meaningful messages), and integrative language functions (i.e., organization of "semantic and symbolic meaning, grammatical structure, and ideas for the production of messages" [WHO, 2001, p. 59]). Abilities related to communication include receiving and producing messages (spoken, nonverbal, written, or formal sign language), carrying on a conversation ("starting, sustaining, and ending a conversation; conversing with one or many people" [WHO, 2001, p. 135]) or discussion ("starting, sustaining, and ending an examination of a matter, with arguments for or against" [WHO, 2001, p. 136], with one or more people), and use of communication devices (e.g., telephones, computers) and techniques (e.g., lip reading) (WHO, 2001). Language and communication are important for the acquisition of mathematical and financial concepts and skills, financial decision making (understanding relevant information and communicating choice), and financial transactions with others.

Summary

The preceding discussion outlines a number of cognitive and behavioral abilities and processes that underlie financial competence. Individuals who are financially competent, in the committee's use of the term, possess the financial knowledge and skills to manage their finances effectively and to make financial decisions and choices that serve their best interests, at least in a controlled setting. Given the broad range of conceptual, procedural, and judgment (decision-making) skills that underlie financial competence, different types and degrees of cognitive impairment will have varying effects on individuals' financial competence (see, e.g., Sherod et al., 2009). Depending on how and to what extent a person's financial competence is affected, he or she may retain financial competence in some areas (e.g., bill paying) but not others (e.g., managing investments). Although such individuals may require assistance in conducting their financial affairs, they nevertheless may be able to direct the management of their funds, as discussed in the following section.

Directing the Management of Funds

Individuals who are financially competent presumably possess the financial knowledge and the conceptual, procedural, and judgment skills required to direct the management of their finances as well as to manage their finances themselves. Nonetheless, financially competent individuals may seek assistance from others in managing their affairs for various reasons, including physical impairments that make it difficult or impossible to complete certain tasks or simply a desire not to complete those tasks themselves because of a lack of time or some other reason. Conversely, people who either do not possess or begin to lose the full complement of cognitive processes and abilities needed for financial competence may still be able to direct the management of their funds.

Various scenarios may arise depending on the areas of cognitive impairment involved. One might retain financial judgment and decision making in terms of making financial choices and setting priorities while having lost the ability to execute such financial tasks as handling money to purchase items (Boyle, 2013). For example, one might know that mortgage, utility, credit card, and other bills must be paid but not be able to keep track of which bills are due when or to execute the steps required to pay them oneself. Alternatively, one might retain the ability to execute day-to-day financial tasks (e.g., transacting purchases, basic banking, bill paying) but have lost the financial judgment skills required for long-term planning or resistance to exploitation or fraud (Marson, 2013).

Some individuals will recognize that they need help and accept or seek out the needed assistance from a family member, friend, community service organization, or other third party. In such cases, the person may be able to direct the management of his or her funds by asking for assistance in the areas in which it is needed while retaining as much control of the funds as possible. In the case of relatively stable conditions (e.g., long-term sequelae of an acquired brain injury or stroke), the person may be able to direct the management of his or her funds indefinitely. On the other hand, in progressive conditions in which the individual's cognitive and behavioral capacities will continue to diminish (e.g., dementia), the person may at some point become unable even to direct the management of his or her funds.

One consideration in determining whether an individual is capable of directing the management of funds is whether the person is capable of appointing a proxy decision maker. Research supports the idea that individuals with dementia, for example, retain the capacity to appoint a proxy to make certain types of decisions even when they have lost the capacity to make those decisions themselves (Kim and Appelbaum, 2006; Kim et al., 2011). Capacity to appoint a proxy to make decisions in a certain area, such as management of one's funds, requires only a general understanding of the nature of the decisions being delegated and trust in someone else to make those decisions (Kim and Appelbaum, 2006). Consistent with the four abilities associated with decision-making capacity, the individual must understand what is at stake in appointing a financial proxy, appreciate how designating such a proxy will affect him or her, indicate a choice about appointing a proxy (or not) and who it should be, and explain the reasoning underlying the choice made (Kim and Appelbaum, 2006).

Even when a proxy has been identified, supported decision making, as discussed in Chapter 3, is one way to preserve an individual's financial autonomy as long as possible or, in some cases, to develop or restore that autonomy. Supported decision making—"the process of providing support to people whose decision making ability is impaired to enable them to make their own decisions wherever possible" (Davidson et al., 2015)—is an important part of a continuum that ranges from independent to substitute decision making. For beneficiaries, supported decision making could entail appointment of a representative payee who receives and has ultimate control over the individual's benefits but who engages the beneficiary in decisions about disbursement of the funds to the extent possible. Such an approach is consistent with SSA's current practice as described in Chapter 2. Alternatively, beneficiaries could receive and have direct control over all or a portion of their benefit payments directly but under the supervision of someone who could assist them with tasks such as budgeting and creating reports to track spending. This approach is consistent with the U.S. Department of Veterans Affairs' (VA's) supervised direct payment program, described in Chapter 2. Another supported decision-making model is the

Advisor Teller Money Manager intervention, a money management-based substance use treatment intervention, in which therapists assist individuals affected by substance use in budgeting their income by having them go to a therapist to access their funds (Rosen et al., 2008, 2010). The therapist helps the clients manage their money, learn to budget their funds, and work to allocate discretionary funds in ways that reinforce constructive activities and limit substance use.

For individuals with a range of disabilities, supported decision making provides the opportunity to receive the assistance they need and want in order to make decisions about their lives, including how their funds are allocated. It is an approach that highlights interdependence as a typical method of decision making—that is, it is rare that any person makes decisions completely independently (United Nations, 2007). Supported decision making allows individuals who need assistance in managing their funds to decide whether they want to participate actively in decision making related to that process and if they do, to provide input on the types of supports they need and prefer.

Unless someone is appointed to assist them, individuals who are able to direct the management of their funds but require assistance in carrying out financial tasks because of physical or cognitive impairments will need to identify an appropriate person or entity to help them. If they cannot locate appropriate third-party assistance, they will be unable to perform financially in the real world even though they are competent to direct the management of their funds. This scenario illustrates one way in which contextual factors—in this case the absence of someone to assist the individual in managing his or her funds—can affect real-world financial performance and why it is important to take such variables into account when assessing an individual's financial capability, as discussed in the following section.

FINANCIAL PERFORMANCE

Performance denotes the actual execution of actions situated in specific contexts and environments (Fisher and Griswold, 2014). How one carries out activities may be learned and developed over time or may be the result of novel or immediate circumstances. Financial performance is affected by factors from several domains, such as financial knowledge, behavior (what a person does with that knowledge), outside influences (factors that contribute to the person's beliefs, attitudes, and behaviors, as well as external supports and barriers), and access (availability and use of appropriate financial products and services) (Sherraden, 2013). Contextual factors can affect an individual's financial performance in the real world negatively or positively. As discussed earlier, individuals who clearly possess financial competence (knowledge and judgment) in a controlled setting (i.e., clearly possess the requisite financial knowledge and conceptual, procedural, and judgment skills to manage their finances successfully) nevertheless may not perform well financially when, for example, they are subjected to real-world temptations (e.g., substance use, addiction disorders, impulse purchases, easy credit). Conversely, individuals with impaired financial knowledge or judgment may perform quite successfully if they have supports in place.

The *ICF* (WHO, 2001, p. 8) conceives of functioning and disability "as a dynamic interaction between health conditions and contextual factors," which include personal and environmental factors. Personal factors are features of an individual that may affect his or her functioning, such as gender, age, social background, education, and past and current experience (WHO, 2001, p. 17). Environmental factors are factors external to individuals that "make up the physical, social, and attitudinal environment in which people live and conduct their lives" (WHO, 2001, p. 16). They include one-time or repeated stressors, social supports, financial and emotional resources, opportunities, and barriers.

Personal Factors

An example of personal factors that affect individuals' financial performance is substance abuse. It impacts financial performance and well-being in a number of ways, including impaired decision making (Bickel et al., 1999; Black and Rosen, 2011; Coffey et al., 2003; Kirby and Petry, 2004; Petry, 2001), increased likelihood of being victimized (Claycomb et al., 2013), failure to maintain stable housing (Drake et al., 1993; Goldfinger et al., 1999; Lipton et al., 2000; North et al., 1998), worsening of psychiatric symptoms and increased risk of hospitalization (Grossman et al., 1997; Rosen et al., 2002; Shaner et al., 1995), and use of benefits to purchase the substances themselves.

Another personal factor that may affect financial performance is one's mental state. Severe depression, for example, may not compromise one's financial competence but may negatively affect one's financial performance. It is important also to take into account fluctuating and fluid capacities and contexts (Lazar et al., 2015a), particularly for those with mental illnesses, as their symptoms, and hence their financial performance, may not remain stable. Changes in medication, medication adherence, and environmental stressors, for example, may alter one's ability to control impulses, manage anxiety, and resist external pressures (Moye et al., 2005).

Religion is another personal factor that may affect decisions about saving and spending money and shape one's ideas about the meaning of money and one's approach to financial management. For example, religious doctrine and thought may emphasize the collective rather than the individual, thus affecting views about the balance of obligations toward oneself and others; specify obligatory family rituals and gift giving; determine one's approach to credit and loans; and so forth (Falicov, 2001). Tithing (i.e., donating a percentage of one's income) to a faith community, for instance, is for some people an important means of fulfilling a religious duty, expressing gratitude, investing in a faith, and promoting social justice and charity. These contributions can constitute a relatively high percentage of one's income (Marks et al., 2009), and thus may alter one's material well-being and entail sacrifices. Religious affiliations and values can lead someone with low income to spend money in ways that may not appear "sound" because they do not always contribute to that individual's financial or material well-being. Unlike other forms of "unsound" spending, however, these expenditures may be intentional, and involve trade-offs that impact spiritual well-being and religious beliefs in a fashion the person deems worthwhile.

Environmental Factors

A number of environmental factors affect not only financial performance but also financial competence. One such factor is socioeconomic status (SES)—a measure of a person's economic and social position in society that is based on wealth, income, education, and occupation (Capuano and Ramsay, 2011; Kehiaian, 2012). SES impacts the opportunity to gain and demonstrate financial knowledge, skills, and behavior, as well as access to financial products and services and resources and opportunities. Worldwide, financial literacy (i.e., knowledge, skills, attitudes, and motivation) is low, and households with low SES demonstrate even lower financial literacy than those with higher SES (Lusardi and Mitchell, 2011). People living in low-income communities typically have less opportunity than their higher-income counterparts to access effective financial instruments (e.g., affordable loans, bank accounts, interest-bearing savings, certificates of deposit) and to gain knowledge of successful financial management principles (i.e., maximizing gains and minimizing losses) (Sherraden, 2013). Conditions of poverty limit people's opportunities to gain knowledge, skills, and behaviors that lead to more effective financial management, such as paying bills on time (Hilgert et al., 2003), having a low-cost bank account (FDIC, 2014), and having emergency savings on hand (Brobeck, 2008).

Research suggests that people gain knowledge as they gain financial experience, and that observed behaviors of their family and friends and economic socialization, as well as resources in their environment, play an important role in shaping their financial knowledge and behaviors (Hilgert et al., 2003; Payne et al., 2014; Sherraden, 2013). People with low income are at a disadvantage in this regard. Many low-income communities, for example, lack convenient access to banks as a result of the consolidation of the banking industry in the past several decades. Moreover, the incessant difficulties resulting from scarce financial resources present cognitive challenges; occupy mental bandwidth; and leave people with less mental capacity for other aspects of everyday life, including some—such as avoiding high-interest loans and remembering to pay bills on time—that are central to successful financial performance (Mullainathan and Shafir, 2013).

People with low income are more likely than those with higher income to be unbanked (i.e., not have a bank account) or underbanked (i.e., have a bank account but also use alternative financial services) (Birkenmaier and Fu, 2015). The alternative financial services to which they tend to have convenient access (e.g., check cashing outlets, payday lenders), increasingly meet the needs of low-income communities for transaction and credit banking services, but at significantly higher costs than those of formal financial institutions (Prager, 2014; Stoesz, 2014).

Limited English proficiency, especially among immigrants to the United States, may further limit access to banks and other traditional financial institutions. Monolingual Spanish-speaking people with low income, in particular, have one of the highest unbanked rates in the nation (FDIC, 2014). Such unbanked households are particularly vulnerable to theft, loss, and debt, and face credit and financial security challenges that go beyond issues of individual financial capability (Morgan-Cross and Klawitter, 2011).

Culture also can affect financial performance. "Economic perspectives are produced through, and situated within, particular sociocultural contexts" (Carpenter-Song, 2012). Cultural understanding of what constitutes appropriate management of one's funds is a product of variations in such factors as people's perceptions of money and resources, locus of control, decision-making patterns, and help-seeking preferences, as well as access to financial knowledge and services. Values, habits, and beliefs concerning how to spend one's money and how to use networks for support are culturally embedded. In some cultures, for example, it may be more important to give money as gifts than to spend money on oneself (Carpenter-Song, 2012). Given local cultural values and beliefs, it can be challenging to distinguish between "extravagance" and "wise spending" (Lazar et al., 2015b; Moye et al., 2005).

Such factors as access to formal bank accounts and financial products, networks of family and friends, the helpfulness of caregivers, opportunities offered by employers, life experiences, the stability and adequacy of living arrangements, real or perceived personal safety, and the quality of financial information available, acting individually or in interaction, can affect a person's financial performance negatively or positively regardless of his or her level of financial competence. For example, people with little financial competence can exhibit positive financial performance with access to (1) helpful family members, friends, or caregivers who educate them about financial matters and help them take advantage of direct deposit of their checks into a low-cost bank account at a formal financial institution (i.e., one that does not charge unreasonable fees for low balances and pays interest); (2) automatic bill paying for basic necessities (e.g., rent, utilities); and (3) a no-fee prepaid debit card with consumer protections to pay for other necessities, such as food. Other salient environmental factors include a stable living environment, experiencing little to no victimization, and few unexpected events that increase expenses and alter one's financial situation. In a study of spouse-carers and individuals with dementia, for example, Boyle (2013) found social factors to be highly important to individuals' financial performance. Those with borderline or diminished capacities could continue participating in making purchases and being engaged in the community given "practical strategies instigated by spouse-carers, such as arranging for purchases to be made on credit" (p. 560). Boyle (2008, 2013) also discusses "assisted autonomy"—strategies that enable people with dementia to utilize their extant capacity and exercise agency. This research highlights the importance of taking noncognitive factors, such as social and emotional supports, into account when assessing and facilitating the financial performance of people with dementia.

Conversely, a person with financial competence may exhibit poor financial performance if he or she (1) receives income through cash or a prepaid card with fees and few or no consumer protections; (2) lacks access to family members, friends, or caregivers who assist with helpful financial information; (3) lacks access to automatic bill paying; (4) lacks access to low-cost, convenient, beneficial financial products and services from a formal financial institution; and (5) lives in a community with conveniently accessed, higher-cost alternative financial services (e.g., check cashers, payday loan stores, auto title companies). The financial performance of a financially competent person also may be negatively affected by residential instability, victimization, and other life experiences (such as a health crisis or loved ones who need cash for their emergencies). Evidence suggests that individuals with the ability to manage their finances may, precisely in contexts of scarcity when careful financial management is critical, show performance difficulties in carrying out those tasks (Shafir, 2015). Emerging literature indicates that the everyday stresses of poverty can make it difficult for people to manage their insufficient resources, avoid highly needed (and often predatory) loans, and resist what may feel like urgent expenditures (Mullainathan and Shafir, 2013).

The Importance of Context

The foregoing discussion makes clear that financial performance is not related solely to an individual's financial competence, but also is affected by the person's context. With supports, individuals with seemingly diminished capacity or judgment may be able to manage their finances effectively. Research in behavioral economics has documented many instances in which small changes in context (e.g., in defaults, in the framing of a problem, in perceived norms) can significantly alter performance (Mullainathan and Shafir, 2013).

To summarize, several types of abilities, including cognitive, perceptual, affective, communicative, and interpersonal, are required for a person to successfully handle the complex demands of managing his or her finances in the context of the challenges, supports, and resources found in his or her environment. These abilities may manifest themselves differently at the levels of competence versus performance. Thus, the person may recognize the need to exercise patience, planning, and impulse control and may even show the requisite abilities in the context of cognitive evaluation in a clinical or laboratory setting, but show diminished financial performance when within an environment rife with fatigue, distraction, stress, and a wide array of temptations. Family and peers, for example, can in some instances provide support and sound advice and in others be a source of stress and bad influence. The abilities necessary to maneuver and succeed in the context of everyday obstacles constitute a level of performance for which a person's competence provides only one ingredient. Conversely, successful performance reflects adequate financial competence (knowledge and judgment), as well as the ability to implement financial decisions in the real world—that is, the presence of sufficient cognitive, perceptual, affective, communicative, and interpersonal abilities to manage or direct others to manage one's benefits. Financial performance is, therefore, the best indicator of financial capability. Figure 1-1 in Chapter 1 illustrates the primacy of evidence of financial performance in determining financial capability.

It is important to note that personal and environmental factors may change or fluctuate, thereby affecting an individual's financial performance. For this reason, it is necessary not only to assess financial performance at a single point in time but also to assess it longitudinally to best estimate a person's financial capability. In addition, interpretations of evidence regarding beneficiaries' financial performance can be informed by evidence of their degree of financial competence.

The committee recognizes that there will be cases in which evidence of real-world financial performance is very limited or unavailable. This may be the case, for example, when the person has had no funds to manage or when no third-party informant with knowledge of the person's performance can be identified. In such cases, evidence of financial competence may be necessary to inform capability determinations. Evidence of financial (in)competence also can help to corroborate, refute, or explain evidence acquired regarding beneficiaries' financial performance.

PREFERENCE FOR PERFORMANCE IN DETERMINING CAPABILITY

The preference for financial performance in determining financial capability is consistent both with the movement toward conceptualizing disability in terms of the interaction between individuals' environment and their functional capacity (IOM, 1991, 1997, 2007; WHO, 2001) and with the reform of guardianship laws in the 1990s (Sabatino and Basinger, 2000).

International Classification of Functioning, Disability and Health (*ICF*) Framework

In 2001, WHO released the *ICF* (WHO, 2001), which was developed through a global consensus-building process. The *ICF* framework (see Figure 4-1) is similar to the conceptual framework used in this report to understand the concept of financial incapability.

The *ICF* framework portrays decrements in human functioning as the product of a dynamic interaction among various health conditions, incapacity to perform specific tasks and actions, and environmental and personal contextual factors that affect human behavior in a real-world context. The *ICF* component that corresponds most closely to the committee's conceptualization of impaired financial performance is *participation*

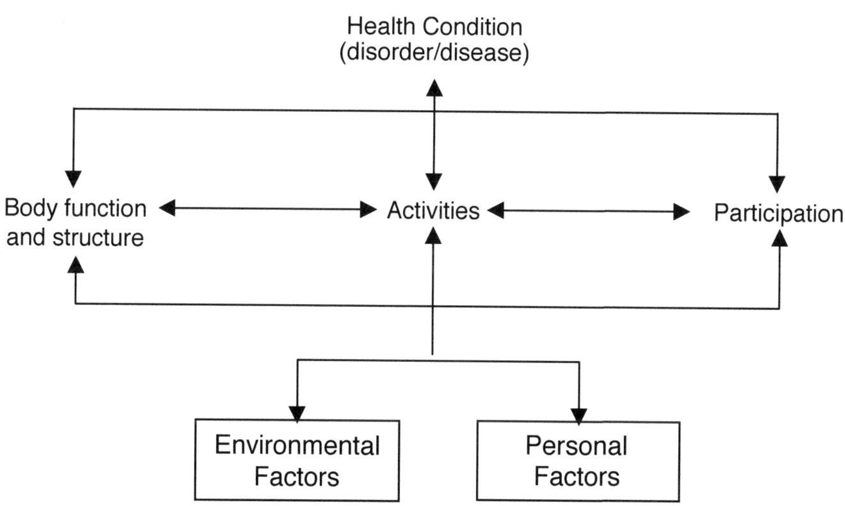

FIGURE 4-1 *International Classification of Functioning, Disability and Health* (*ICF*) framework.
SOURCE: WHO, 2001, p. 18.

restriction, defined as "problems an individual may experience in involvement in life situations" (WHO, 2001, p. 10). Restriction is explained as the "discordance between the observed and expected performance," where expected performance refers to a "population norm" or standard based on the "experience of people without the specific health condition" (p. 15). Performance is described as "what an individual does in his or her current environment." This is in contrast to the *ICF* concept of *activity limitation*, which denotes limits on a person's ability to execute a task or action—similar to the committee's concept of financial competence.

The *ICF* framework includes the concept of a *health condition*, a general term for a disease, disorder, injury, trauma, congenital anomaly, or genetic characteristic, the starting point for subsequent development of *activity limitation* and/or *participation restriction* (WHO, 2001). As with the conceptual model for the present report, the *ICF* includes environmental and personal factors as mediating contextual elements. *Environmental factors* are "all aspects of the external or extrinsic world" that form "the physical, social, and attitudinal circumstances in which people live and conduct their lives" (WHO, 2001, pp. 10, 213). *Personal factors* include gender, race, age, coping styles, and other individual characteristics that are not classified in the *ICF*. These contextual factors may act as facilitators or barriers as they affect a person's activity or participation, much as contextual factors, such as those described in the previous section, can influence a person's financial performance.

Reforms in Guardianship Law

Guardianship law specifies criteria for a legal determination that an individual is unable to make decisions about his or her person or property and that the state may therefore limit the person's autonomy and appoint a guardian to protect his or her interests. The criteria for establishing legal incapacity are subject to change based on the "prevailing values, knowledge, and even the economic and political spirit of the time" (Sabatino and Basinger, 2000, p. 121). In the United States, guardianship laws and the criteria they embody have evolved over time. The early laws established determinations based on labels (e.g., "lunatic," "person of unsound mind") or behavior (e.g., excessive drinking, gambling, debauchery). Over time, most states adopted a medical approach that included requiring the presence of one or more disabling conditions, often specifying that the conditions "must result in a functional impairment with respect to one's *ability to manage his or her property or person*" (Sabatino and Basinger, 2000, p. 123). Gradually, states began to replace that type of broad functional behavior test first with a more specific criterion focused on one's ability to meet essential needs, such as food, shelter, and safety, and later with a cognitive functioning test. In addition, some states dropped the disabling condition requirement. Although the 1982 Uniform Guardianship and Protective Proceedings Act retained the disabling condition requirement, it included a test of cognitive functioning. In 1997, the act was revised to remove the disabling condition requirement and incorporate an essential needs standard into the test of cognitive functioning (Sabatino and Basinger, 2000, pp. 126-127):

> "Incapacitated person" means an individual who, for reasons other than being a minor, is unable to receive and evaluate information or make or communicate decisions to such an extent that the individual lacks the ability to meet essential requirements for physical health, safety, or self-care, even with appropriate technological assistance. (National Conference of Commissioners on Uniform State Laws, 1997, sec. 102)

The committee's preference for a performance-based standard for making determinations of financial capability is consistent with the movement in U.S. guardianship law away from a standard focused on an individual's medical condition to one focused on a person's functional ability to meet basic needs. It also is consistent with the *ICF* framework, which emphasizes real-world functioning (performance) that stems from a complex interplay among an individual's health conditions, abilities (competence), and contextual factors. Both the evolution of guardianship law and the development of the *ICF* provide context and support for the committee's emphasis on financial performance in capability determinations.

MENTAL AND PHYSICAL DISORDERS THAT MAY AFFECT FINANCIAL CAPABILITY

SSA asked the committee to identify specific mental and physical disorders, such as those in SSA's *Listing of Impairments* for adults [Part A] (SSA, n.d.-b) or in SSA's adult Compassionate Allowances templates (SSA, n.d.-a), that by definition preclude capability or that strongly indicate incapability. SSA also requested that the committee identify any mental or physical disorders for which the determination of capability could be made based solely on objective medical evidence.[6] While believing that the best

[6] In SSA terms, *objective medical evidence* refers to medical signs and laboratory findings. Laboratory findings must be demonstrated through "medically acceptable laboratory diagnostic techniques," among which SSA includes psychological tests (20 CFR § 404.1528). "Signs are anatomical, physiological, or psychological abnormalities which can be observed, apart from [self-reported symptoms]. Signs must be shown by medically acceptable clinical diagnostic techniques. Psychiatric signs are medically demonstrable phenomena that indicate specific psychological abnormalities, e.g., abnormalities of behavior, mood, thought, memory, orientation, development, or perception. They must also be shown by observable facts that can be medically described and evaluated" (20 CFR § 404.1528). "Laboratory findings are anatomical, physiological, or psychological phenomena which can be shown by the use of medically acceptable laboratory diagnostic techniques. Some of these diagnostic techniques

indicators of financial capability are actual knowledge of individuals' functional performance in their everyday environments and their consistency[7] in managing financial matters and making financial decisions that are in their self-interest, the committee appreciates the expediency of a list of mental and physical conditions that preclude capability or that strongly indicate incapability. For a variety of reasons, however, the committee notes that there exist only a very limited number of conditions whose presence can be the sole basis for a capability determination.

To qualify for disability benefits under the Supplemental Security Income or Social Security Disability Insurance program, an applicant must have a physical or mental impairment severe in nature and of such duration that the person is unable to participate in any substantial gainful activity (Wixon and Strand, 2013). A medically determinable physical or mental impairment or combination of impairments is considered severe "if it significantly limits an individual's physical or mental abilities to do basic work activities" (SSA, 1996). SSA's *Listing of Impairments* "describes, for each major body system, impairments considered severe enough to prevent an individual from doing any gainful activity" (SSA, n.d.-c). "Most of the listed impairments are permanent or expected to result in death, or the listing includes a specific statement of duration. For all other listings, the evidence must show that the impairment has lasted or is expected to last for a continuous period of at least 12 months" (SSA, n.d.-c). The *Listing of Impairments* is organized by major body system and contains criteria for evaluating the severity of a listed impairment. These criteria may include assessments of work-related functioning[8] and are designed to identify individuals with impairments that are sufficiently severe to prohibit them from engaging in any kind of "gainful activity" (SSA, n.d.-c). In some cases, an individual has multiple impairments, none of which is, by itself, sufficiently severe to meet the *Listing* criteria, or an impairment that is not included in the *Listing*. In such cases, the examiner considers whether the impairment or combination of impairments is medically equal to a listed impairment. If an otherwise qualified applicant's impairment(s) meets or equals the *Listing* criteria, the claim is allowed.[9]

SSA recognizes that some conditions are so severe that they obviously meet its disability standards. The Compassionate Allowances initiative

---

include chemical tests, electrophysiological studies (electrocardiogram, electroencephalogram, etc.), roentgenological studies (X-rays), and psychological tests" (20 CFR § 404.1528).

[7] *Consistency* in this context means the individual behaves in a manner that adheres to the same or similar principles and intentions across time and situations.

[8] For mental disorders, functional limitations are used to assess the severity of the impairment. Paragraph B and C criteria in the *Listing of Impairments* for mental disorders describe the areas of function that are considered necessary for work (SSA, n.d.-d).

[9] All remaining applications move on to the next step in the disability evaluation process.

allows SSA to quickly identify applicants who invariably will qualify for disability benefits under the *Listing of Impairments* based on objective medical information that it can obtain quickly (SSA, n.d.-a).

In the following section, the committee discusses mental disorders and physical conditions that affect individuals' cognitive and behavioral capacities and considers whether any of them would categorically preclude financial capability or strongly indicate incapability. In the subsequent section, the committee considers the same questions with respect to physical disorders that do not directly affect an individual's cognitive capacity.

Disorders with Cognitive Effects

Evaluation of financial capability is important in individuals who have disorders that are severe enough to lead to work-related disability and negatively affect the cognitive domains relevant to financial competence discussed earlier—namely, general cognitive/intellectual ability, attention and vigilance, learning and memory, executive function, social cognition, and language and communication. Although the presence of such disorders raises the need for assessment of financial capability, their diagnosis alone ordinarily is not sufficient for making a capability determination. One difficulty is the variable impact of disorders on the individuals affected; another is the lack of correlation in many cases between the severity of one's clinical symptoms and one's functional limitations.

SSA's evaluation of disability on the basis of mental disorders requires not only documentation of a medically determinable impairment(s) but also consideration of the degree of limitation imposed by the impairment(s) on the applicant's ability to work, as well as whether these limitations have lasted or are expected to last for a continuous period of at least 12 months (SSA, n.d.-d). SSA's *Listing of Impairments* for adults, Section 12.00, "Mental Disorders," is arranged in nine diagnostic categories: organic mental disorders (12.02); schizophrenic, paranoid, and other psychotic disorders (12.03); affective disorders (12.04); intellectual disability (12.05); anxiety-related disorders (12.06); somatoform disorders (12.07); personality disorders (12.08); substance addiction disorders (12.09); and autistic disorder and other pervasive developmental disorders (12.10).

> For most of the diagnostic categories,[10] adult applicants will meet a listing if the impairment satisfies the following: (1) the diagnostic description

[10] The structure of the listings for intellectual disability and for substance addiction disorders differs from that of the other mental disorder listings. There are four sets of criteria (Paragraphs A through D) for the intellectual disability listing, and the listing for substance addiction disorders refers to which of the other listings should be used to evaluate the various physical or behavioral changes related to the disorder.

> of the mental disorder; (2) specified medical findings—e.g., symptoms (self-report), signs (medically demonstrable), laboratory findings (including psychological test findings)—(Paragraph A criteria); and (3) specified "impairment-related functional limitations that are incompatible with the ability to do any gainful activity" (Paragraph B or Paragraph C criteria) (SSA, n.d.-d). Paragraph A criteria, in conjunction with the diagnostic description, substantiate the presence of the specific mental disorder based on the medical evidence. Paragraph B and Paragraph C criteria list the functional limitations resulting from the mental impairment that preclude the ability to engage in gainful activity. (IOM, 2015, p. 53)[11]

Many of the conditions that fall into these mental disorder diagnostic categories raise concern about an individual's ability to manage his or her finances. Other conditions also may cause symptoms that include cognitive effects. For example, disorders associated with severe, unremitting pain (e.g., cancer metastatic to the bones), extreme debilitation (e.g., metastatic cancer, advanced heart failure), hypoxia (e.g., severe obstructive lung disease), and endocrine and metabolic imbalances (e.g., thyrotoxicosis, Addison's disease, hyponatremia, hyperparathyroidism), as well as certain neurological conditions (e.g., Huntington's disease, Parkinson's disease), can affect the capacities relevant to financial capability. The following sections address several broad types of disorders that may impair financial capability, including neurocognitive disorders, such as dementias; neurodevelopmental disorders; psychiatric disorders; substance-related disorders; and traumatic brain injury (TBI).

Neurocognitive Disorders

Neurocognitive disorders, which encompass SSA's Listing 12.02 (organic mental disorders), include disorders of the brain, such as Alzheimer's disease, diffuse Lewy body disease, frontotemporal dementia (e.g., Pick's disease), vascular dementia, multiple system atrophy, and progressive supranuclear palsy, that are associated with cognitive decline (American Psychiatric Association, 2013). In addition, some neurological disorders, such as Huntington's disease or Parkinson's disease, may progress to result in dementia and decline in cognitive domains. Individuals who are diagnosed with moderate or severe stages of these types of disease typically experience so many difficulties with cognitive function and orientation to time, place, and person, as well as with judgment, that they are unable to carry out many activities of daily living, including management of finances. They frequently require another person to help them with these activities and would be in danger without these supports. Furthermore,

[11] This text has been modified from the prepublication version of the report.

most of these conditions are degenerative; that is, they are characterized by worsening over time. Studies of individuals with Alzheimer's disease using the Financial Capacity Instrument (Griffith et al., 2003; Marson et al., 2000) indicate that impairment of financial competence appears first in mild cognitive impairment, is already widespread in people with mild Alzheimer's disease, and is advanced and global in those with moderate levels of such disease (Griffith et al., 2003; Marson et al., 2000; Stoeckel et al., 2013; Triebel et al., 2009).

The *Listing of Impairments* takes account of the severity of applicants' impairments with respect to their ability to perform gainful activity. Paragraph B criteria focus on functional limitations in four areas: (1) activities of daily living; (2) social functioning; (3) concentration, persistence, or pace; and (4) episodes of decompensation. To meet the Paragraph B criteria for organic mental disorders, the impairment as specified must result in at least two of the following: (1) marked restriction of activities of daily living; (2) marked difficulties in maintaining social functioning; (3) marked difficulties in maintaining concentration, persistence, or pace; or (4) repeated episodes of decompensation, each of extended duration (SSA, n.d.-e). "Marked" means more than moderate but less than extreme. A marked limitation is one in which "the degree of limitation is such as to interfere seriously with [one's] ability to function independently, appropriately, effectively, and on a sustained basis (SSA, n.d.-d; see also §§ 404.1520a and 416.920a). Although someone who qualified for disability by meeting the *Listing* criteria for organic mental disorder might be incapable of managing or directing the management of his or her finances, the disability determination process focuses on individuals' work-related impairment for the purpose of determining whether they qualify to receive benefits. The impairment threshold for determining disability may reasonably differ from that required to justify interference with beneficiaries' autonomy with respect to management of their disability payment. As discussed in Chapter 3, the decision to appoint a representative payee must entail weighing the beneficiary's personal autonomy and preferences against interventions that, while infringing on the beneficiary's autonomy, are meant to protect his or her best interests. Deeming an adult to be incapable when he or she is not erodes personal liberty, establishes stigma through labeling, leaves the individual open to exploitation, and deprives the person of the freedom to direct personally appropriate actions based on long-held values and preferences. It therefore is reasonable to require a higher threshold of cognitive impairment for capability determination than for disability determination. For this reason, it would be imprudent to attempt to map the level of impairment associated with financial incompetence onto the level of impairment for work-related disability contained in the *Listing of Impairments*.

There are other difficulties as well with relying solely on diagnosis and medical evidence in making determinations of financial capability. One is the variable impact of disorders on the individuals affected; as noted earlier, different people experience and respond to medical conditions differently. Another is the lack of correlation in many cases between the severity of one's clinical symptoms and one's functional limitations. In addition, people may experience variations in their symptoms over time—especially earlier in the course of the illness—such as the fluctuations in cognition, either above or below baseline, that have been observed in people with different types of dementia (Lee et al., 2012). Fluctuations reflecting improved function have been associated with the legal concept of the lucid interval, which refers to a discrete, temporary period of time during which an otherwise incompetent individual is found to have the requisite capacity to execute a valid will (Shulman et al., 2015). However, the developing medical literature on cognitive fluctuation raises questions about the validity of the concept of a lucid interval (Shulman et al., 2015). Specifically, the fluctuations often are of short duration (i.e., seconds or minutes) and are relatively minor (e.g., an improvement over the person's current baseline rather than to his or her predisease state of lucidity). In addition, the fluctuations affect primarily alertness and attention rather than memory and executive function, which are also important for financial competence (Shulman et al., 2015). At the same time, it should be noted that the nature of these fluctuations differs among types of dementia. In particular, studies have found fluctuations reflecting decrements in cognition in dementia with Lewy bodies to be associated primarily with decreased awareness and attention, while in Alzheimer's dementia they are associated more with impaired memory (Bradshaw et al., 2004; Lee et al., 2012). Also, the fluctuations in the former condition appear to be more frequent, shorter in duration, and more intense than those observed in the latter (Bradshaw et al., 2004; Lee et al., 2012). In contrast to fluctuating cognition in Alzheimer's disease, cognitive fluctuations in dementia with Lewy bodies often reflect transient decrements in function, followed by return to a near-normal level of cognitive function (Bradshaw et al., 2004), suggesting that such individuals may retain their financial capability some or most of the time even if they experience transient periods of financial incompetence. Finally, as previously discussed, contextual factors also may support continued successful financial performance in individuals experiencing a level of cognitive impairment sufficient to qualify for SSA disability benefits.

For all of these reasons, diagnosis and medical evidence of impairment alone constitute an insufficient basis for making determinations of financial capability in all but the most severe cases. It is important to note, however, that given the progressive nature of dementias, once an individual with dementia is no longer able to manage or direct the management of his or her finances, the expectation is that the ability to do so will not return. Similarly, individuals with dementia who are still able to manage or direct the management of their finances are expected to lose that ability as their condition progresses and will need to be reevaluated on a regular basis.

Neurodevelopmental Disorders

The presence of neurodevelopmental disorders such as intellectual disability (Listing 12.05) and autistic disorder and other pervasive developmental disorders (Listing 12.10) also signals the need to evaluate individuals' financial capability. As noted in Chapter 1, SSA generally presumes that adult beneficiaries are financially capable absent evidence to the contrary. One exception is beneficiaries who meet mental disorder listing for intellectual disability 12.05A or 12.05B (SSA, n.d.-f). Individuals who qualify for disability under 12.05A demonstrate "mental incapacity evidenced by dependence upon others for personal needs (e.g., toileting, eating, dressing, or bathing) and inability to follow directions, such that the use of standardized measures of intellectual functioning is precluded." Individuals who qualify for disability under 12.05B are those who possess "a valid verbal, performance, or full scale IQ [intelligence quotient] of 59 or less" (SSA, n.d.-f).

It appears clear that individuals who are sufficiently intellectually impaired so as not to be testable using standardized measures of intellectual functioning will also be financially incapable and will require a representative payee. The situation with respect to individuals who have a valid verbal, performance, or full-scale IQ of 59 or less is more complicated.

A small study of individuals with a mean full-scale IQ of 59 (range 50-67) showed performance on a temporal discounting task and a financial decision-making task to be related more strongly to executive functioning than to IQ (Willner et al., 2010a). In the first task, participants were asked to make a series of choices between smaller, more immediate rewards and larger, delayed rewards. The second task presented a series of increasingly complex scenarios in which a choice had to be made. For each scenario, the participants were asked a series of questions to elucidate their performance on five aspects of decision making (identification, understanding, reasoning, appreciation, and communication). Decision making on both tasks (temporal decision making and financial decision making) was based primarily on a single class of information (e.g., delay in reward, amount of reward) rather than a weighing of multiple pieces of information. This suggests that weighing different pieces of information for the purpose of decision making may be problematic for individuals with the participants' level of intellectual disability. However, the association between difficulties with weighing multiple sources of information and executive function rather than IQ suggests the possible benefit of psychoeducational strategies in improving decision making (Willner et al., 2010a). It also supports the view that functional assessment of financial performance is a better indicator of financial capability than IQ alone. A study of participants with a mean full-scale IQ of less than 70 (standard deviation [SD] = 5.4) generated similar results. That study found performance on a temporal discounting task among individuals with intellectual disability to be random, and when respondents' choices were nonrandom (i.e., consistent), they displayed impulsivity. The study also showed that training improved the consistency of decision making among participants and that both initial and post-training performance were related to executive functioning rather than to IQ (Willner et al., 2010b).

The same group also looked at basic financial knowledge (versus understanding or functional ability) in participants with a mean full-scale IQ of 59.1 (SD = 5.1) (Willner et al., 2011). The test comprised a coin recognition task and a cost identification task (estimating the cost of certain items). Most participants identified all of the coins and the cost of an ice cream, but identification of costs for other, more expensive, items was poor. The total scores were significantly correlated "with receptive language ability and performance on memory tests but not with IQ or executive functioning" (Willner et al., 2011, p. 285).

A small study of men and women with a mean full-scale IQ of 61.8 (SD = 10.59) examined their financial decision-making abilities through the use of vignettes and semistructured interviews and compared the results with those obtained from two comparison groups (Suto et al., 2005a). Although the financial decision-making abilities of the participants with mild intellectual disability generally were found to be weaker than those of participants in the "general population" and "very able" comparison groups, individual scores varied widely, and many individuals with mild intellectual disability were judged capable of making at least some personal financial decisions. For some decisions, certain participants with intellectual disability scored higher than several individuals in the comparison groups. Participants in all three groups had the most difficulty with understanding and reasoning with the information relevant to the decision. The results of this study indicate that the financial decision-making processes across all three groups were not qualitatively different and that decision-making abilities exist along a continuum. Although the abilities relate broadly to tested intellectual ability, there is no perfect correlation, and other factors must be involved. The authors conclude that the findings support a functional approach to the assessment of financial decision making for both legal and clinical purposes.

A second analysis of data from the same participants identified correlations among financial decision-making abilities, intellectual ability, understanding of some basic concepts relevant to finance, and decision-making opportunities in everyday life (Suto et al., 2005b). The analysis indicated a direct relationship between intellectual disability and basic financial understanding, but also found "strong relationships of a potentially reciprocal nature between basic financial understanding and everyday decision-making opportunities and between such opportunities and financial decision-making abilities" (Suto et al., 2005b, p. 210). The findings of this study suggest that access to basic skills education and to everyday decision-making opportunities are both critically important to the development of financial decision-making ability, which intellectual ability plays only an indirect role in determining (Suto et al., 2005b).

A third study by the same group (Suto et al., 2006) used five measures entailing identification and ordering tasks to examine understanding of quantity, numbers, and money. The authors found that the concept of quantity was easier to understand than the concepts of numbers and money, with individual performance on tasks decreasing as the magnitudes of numbers and money involved in the tasks increased. The authors conclude that the measures examined may help inform interventions to maximize independent financial decision making (Suto et al., 2006).

Autism spectrum disorder (ASD) is a lifelong condition characterized by persistent deficits in social communication and social interaction across multiple contexts and restricted, repetitive patterns of behavior, interests, or activities (American Psychiatric Association, 2013). Because ASD is a spectrum disorder, the symptoms, intellectual ability, and functional skills of those affected vary widely. Recent research indicates that adults with ASD often have significant deficits in the area of daily living skills, which include using money, banking, and managing finances (Matthews et al., 2015; Smith et al., 2012). One study found that adults with ASD failed to perform more than one-third of daily living skills as measured on the Waisman Activities of Daily Living Scale (Smith et al., 2012). Matthews and colleagues (2015) report that, although a relative strength, standard scores on the Daily Living Domain of the Vineland Adaptive Behavior Scale were on average below 70 in adults with ASD, indicating a significant deficit. To date, no studies have looked specifically at financial management in adults with ASD. Findings of the available research, however, suggest that adults with ASD with severe intellectual disabilities are likely to need supports for carrying out daily living skills, including managing finances.

Determining financial capability in adults with ASD without intellectual disabilities or with mild forms of these disabilities may be more challenging as symptoms and skills in these cases vary widely. Many adults with ASD have significant gaps between their intellectual ability and daily living skills; that is, their IQ scores may be in the average range and their daily living scores well below average (Duncan and Bishop, 2013). A range of factors, including deficits in executive function (Gilloty et al., 2002), social cognition (Eack et al., 2013), and social judgment (Forgeot d'Arc et al., 2014), may influence the ability of an adult with ASD to manage his or her finances.

Psychiatric Disorders

Chronic schizophrenia, paranoia, and other psychotic disorders (Listing 12.03) are characterized by psychotic features with deterioration from a previous level of functioning. Other conditions also can cause cognitive and functional impairments, requiring careful investigation into the need for a representative payee. Examples include bipolar disorder (affective disorders [Listing 12.04]); major depressive disorder; and substance use disorders (substance addiction disorders [Listing 12.09]), discussed in the following section. In research, the topic of financial capacity in individuals with serious mental illnesses such as schizophrenia and bipolar disorder has received little attention compared with such topics as the capacity to provide informed consent to treatment or research participation (Marson et al., 2006).

A small Japanese study of individuals diagnosed with schizophrenia examined financial competence and its relationship to cognitive function using the Financial Competency Assessment Tool (FCAT), developed by Sakuraba and colleagues (2004) for assessing multiple domains of financial competence based on task performance in persons with mental illness, and the Japanese version of the Neurobehavioral Cognitive Status Examination (COGNISTAT) (Niekawa et al., 2007). The FCAT assesses financial competence in six domains: basic monetary skills, financial conceptual knowledge, utilization of a banking institution, cash transaction, financial judgment, and understanding own income and expenditures. Each domain is scored, and the total FCAT score (range 0-37) is used as a global measure of financial competence, with 20/21 set as the cut-off for "distinguishing independence of money management in daily life" (Sakuraba et al., 2004). The individuals with schizophrenia performed significantly worse than the comparison group on tasks in all domains of the FCAT, and a significantly greater number of those in the former group scored below the cut-off point (Niekawa et al., 2007).

The problems the FCAT demonstrated in the schizophrenia group may be related to impairment of several cognitive functions, in particular comprehension and constructional abilities, as assessed on the COGNISTAT battery. Barrett and colleagues (2009) examined the financial skills of 49 outpatients diagnosed with schizophrenia or schizoaffective disorder compared with a comparison group with no history of mental illness.

The outpatient group included both individuals who had either a court-appointed guardian or a representative payee (n = 24) (financially dependent group) and those who managed their finances independently (n = 25) (financially independent group). All participants were aged 55 or younger, had no diagnosed dementia or mental retardation, had an IQ of 70 or greater (based on the reading test of the Wide Range Achievement Test-Revised), and had no history of head injury with loss of consciousness for more than 30 minutes (Barrett et al., 2009). The study found that the financially dependent group scored significantly worse than the financially independent and comparison groups on the financial skills subscale of the Direct Assessment of Functional Status, with a lower percentage of the dependent group receiving a passing score. The financially independent and comparison groups did not differ significantly (Barrett et al., 2009). The findings of this study indicate that some individuals with schizophrenia or schizoaffective disorder can manage their finances independently, while others require a representative payee. The authors are silent on whether they controlled for substance (ab)use among participants.

Bipolar disorder is frequently associated with impulsivity (Najt et al., 2007), including impulsive spending (DiNicola et al., 2010). In a study of 158 individuals diagnosed with bipolar disorder, 33 percent demonstrated at least one behavioral addiction, compared with 13 percent of the comparison group. The individuals with bipolar disorder scored significantly higher than the comparison group on the scales for pathological gambling ($p < 0.001$), compulsive buying ($p < 0.05$), and other addictive behaviors (DiNicola et al., 2010). These findings suggest the potential for money mismanagement and the need to evaluate for financial capability in individuals with bipolar disorder, although the committee is unaware of studies examining financial capability per se in these individuals.

In the vast majority of cases, diagnosis of a psychiatric disorder alone is insufficient evidence with which to render a decision regarding the need for a representative payee, and an assessment of the individual's financial capability is required. One of the challenges in assessing financial capability in persons with certain psychiatric disorders is the fluctuations in the presence, severity, and nature of symptoms noted earlier. Some people with bipolar disorder may lack financial capability during manic episodes but possess that capability during periods of stable mood. Similarly, individuals with schizophrenia typically experience exacerbations of symptoms (often referred to as "decompensation"), during which psychotic symptoms, conceptual disorganization, and/or behavioral symptoms worsen and lead to increased functional impairment. In some of these cases, a determination of financial capability made at one point in time may not be valid when the person is decompensating.

Substance Use and Addiction Disorders

Although substance use *by itself* is neither a qualifying condition for SSA disability nor grounds for a determination of incapability to manage SSA benefits, substance use and addiction, as well as behavioral addictions such as compulsive gambling, can cause individuals who may display financial competence in an office or clinical setting to perform poorly (exercise poor financial judgment) in the real world. This is an important consideration given the frequent comorbidity of substance (ab)use in individuals with psychotic and affective disorders (Frank and Degan, 1997; Regier et al., 1990; Rosen et al., 2002; Shaner et al., 1995).

Studies indicate a relationship between drug and alcohol use disorders and a demonstrated preference of users for immediate rewards that are temporary or less valuable over delayed but sustainable or more valuable rewards (Bickel et al., 1999; Black and Rosen, 2011; Coffey et al., 2003; Kirby and Petry, 2004; Petry, 2001). Substance abuse also is associated with increased risk for housing insecurity and homelessness (Drake et al., 1993; Olfson et al., 1999). Substance abuse is often the proximate cause of an episode of homelessness, and results of several studies suggest that relapse to substance use is the most important personal factor leading to homelessness among previously housed people with psychiatric illness (Goldfinger et al., 1999; Lipton et al., 2000). An analysis of data on 900 homeless persons found a pattern of progressing from an initial diagnosis of psychiatric illness to later substance abuse and homelessness (North et al., 1998).

Financial victimization is more likely among people with recent substance use. A study of 122 adult recipients of SSA disability payments who were receiving inpatient or intensive outpatient psychiatric treatment included assessments of money management and financial victimization (Claycomb et al., 2013). Fully 70 percent of the respondents reported experiencing financial victimization in the preceding 28 days. Financial victimization occurred more frequently among those who had used alcohol more during this period, were younger, and had more frequent psychiatric hospitalizations. Difficulty managing money was most strongly associated with financial victimization.

A Swiss study of 57 individuals diagnosed with schizophrenia showed that they spent as much as 47 percent of their discretionary money on addictive substances (cigarettes, alcohol, cannabis) (Borras et al., 2007). The percentage of discretionary funds thus expended ranged from 24 percent among individuals living with family members (n = 12), to 36 percent among those living alone (n = 15), to 47 percent among those living in supported housing (n = 30).

Other studies have shown that substance use linked with receipt of monthly disability checks can lead to exhaustion of funds needed to meet basic needs, exacerbation of psychiatric symptoms, and hospital admissions (Grossman et al., 1997; Rosen et al., 2002; Shaner et al., 1995). Shaner and colleagues (1995), for example, found that cocaine use, psychiatric symptoms, and hospital admissions among 105 men with schizophrenia and long-term cocaine dependence peaked shortly after the arrival of their disability payment on the first day of each month. The authors also found that the average participant in the study spent nearly half his total income on illegal drugs. They conclude that "the consequences of this cycle include the depletion of funds needed for housing and food, exacerbation of psychiatric symptoms, more frequent psychiatric hospitalization, and a high rate of homelessness" (Shaner et al., 1995).

A study of 236 psychiatric inpatients at four VA hospitals evaluated the relationship between substance abuse and clinician-rated need for assistance with money management. The study found that (1) severity of alcohol and drug use was modestly associated with the need for assistance, (2) the effect of severity of substance use was greater in patients with coexisting major mental illness, and (3) only severity of drug use was significantly associated with the need for a payee (Rosen et al., 2002).

Traumatic Brain Injury

Severe TBI can render individuals incapable of the financial knowledge or judgment necessary to fulfill their interests in the everyday environment. Claimants who are in a coma for at least 30 days are automatically presumed incapable (SSA, 2015a). Although individuals in a coma clearly lack financial capability at that time, with the return of consciousness their condition can evolve to the point that their capability to manage or direct the management of their benefits is restored. Periodic reassessment of the status of these individuals is therefore important to determine whether and to what extent they have recovered. Short of coma, neuropsychological assessment is necessary to determine the severity and expected course of cognitive dysfunction resulting from TBI, as is assessment to determine financial capability.

A small study of individuals with moderate to severe TBI found multiple cognitive functions to be associated with initial impairment and partial recovery of financial competence (which the authors refer to as "capacity"). Participants with moderate to severe TBI and a sample of adult comparison subjects were administered the Financial Capacity Instrument (FCI-9) for assessment of financial skills and abilities at baseline (30 days postinjury for the TBI group) and at a 6-month follow-up visit (Dreer et al., 2012; Martin et al., 2012). Mental arithmetic/working memory and immediate verbal memory were key cognitive functions predicting FCI performance a month following injury ($R^2 = 0.72$, $p < 0.001$) (Martin et al., 2012). Six months following injury, however, executive function and mental arithmetic/working memory were key cognitive functions mediating FCI performance ($R^2 = 0.79$, $p < 0.001$) (Martin et al., 2012). Executive function and mental arithmetic/working memory also were the best baseline predictors of FCI performance in participants with TBI at 6-month follow-up ($R^2 = 0.71$, $p < 0.001$) (Martin et al., 2012). Findings from this study highlight the importance of arithmetic, working memory, and executive function skills in the recovery of financial competence in individuals with moderate to severe TBI.

Another study with the same sample found that individuals with moderate to severe TBI showed improvement in both simple and complex financial skills over a 6-month period. Baseline assessment 30 days post-injury showed that the participants with TBI performed significantly below the level of the comparison group in simple and complex financial skills, suggesting that a marked loss of financial abilities occurred immediately following injury (Dreer et al., 2012). At the 6-month follow-up, however, participants with TBI demonstrated notable improvement in both simple and complex financial skills (Dreer et al., 2012). These findings show the importance of periodic reassessment and the use of strategies that can help individuals with moderate to severe TBI regain critical skills in the acute rehabilitation setting. Despite notable improvement at the 6-month follow-up, participants with TBI remained impaired in complex financial domains such as financial concepts, checkbook management, and bill payment, thus showing only a partial improvement in financial capacity (Dreer et al., 2012). These findings have important implications. Immediately following moderate to severe TBI, most individuals are unable to manage finances and need education and support from a family member who can assume those functions for them. Health care providers also can provide guidance to individuals with TBI and their family members regarding the need for immediate support following the injury and continued support on complex financial tasks.

Summary

Although the committee takes the position that financial performance is the most important consideration in making a determination of financial capability, there are several classes of mental conditions that by their nature make it likely that the affected individual will need a representative payee now or in the future. In particular, the presence of certain mental disorders severe enough to lead to work disability—such as a well-documented history of severe intellectual disability; significant autism; or advanced Alzheimer's disease, frontotemporal dementia, or dementia with Lewy bodies—may be sufficient for a determination of incapability. Such examples are in a minority, however, because there are milder forms or stages of these conditions, as well as psychiatric conditions such as bipolar disorder or substance use disorders, characterized by waxing and waning of symptoms. For these cases, determinations of financial capability are much more complex. Therefore, diagnostic classifications alone are inferior to actual knowledge of individuals' functional performance in their everyday environments and their consistency in managing financial matters and making financial decisions that are in their self-interest.

Disorders with No or Minimal Cognitive Effects

The *Listing of Impairments* for adults also includes physical disorders or impairments. Physical disorders, such as certain neurodegenerative disorders, that may entail an element of cognitive impairment are discussed in the previous section. This section focuses solely on disorders that do not directly affect an individual's cognitive capacity. Although cognitively capable individuals with certain disorders may require and arrange for assistance to accomplish the physical tasks necessary to manage their benefits, they retain the capability to direct others to manage their benefits for them. They therefore are financially capable despite their physical limitations.

Exceptions to this observation are the very few physical impairments that completely preclude communication with others to direct the management of benefits even with the use of assistive communication devices. Examples include myopathies (e.g., mitochondrial myopathies) and neuromuscular disorders (e.g., advanced ALS [amyotrophic lateral sclerosis] or locked-in syndrome) of such severity that any form of communication has become impossible.

SUMMARY

This chapter has elaborated on the concepts of *financial competence* (*financial knowledge* and *financial judgment*) and *financial performance* as defined by the committee. The declarative and procedural knowledge and decision-making abilities necessary for financial competence, along with the relevant cognitive domains, have been described. An individual's financial competence may be demonstrated through assigned tasks in a clinical or office setting. By contrast, financial performance refers to one's degree of success in handling financial demands in the real world. Although successful financial performance reflects sufficient financial competence to implement financial decisions in the real world, a variety of personal and environmental contextual factors can improve or diminish an individual's real-world financial performance. For this reason, the committee concludes that financial performance is the best indicator of financial capability. The committee's preference for financial performance in determining financial capability is consistent both with the movement toward conceptualizing disability in terms of the interaction between individuals' environment and their functional capacity and with the reform of guardianship laws in the 1990s. Because personal and environmental factors may change or fluctuate, thereby affecting an individual's financial performance, it is necessary to assess it across time to best estimate a person's financial capability.

The committee recognizes that there will be times when no or very limited information is available about a beneficiary's financial performance—for example, when the person has had no funds to manage or when no third-party informant with knowledge of the person's performance can be identified. When evidence of financial performance is unavailable, evidence of financial competence may need to be used to inform capability determinations. Evidence of beneficiaries' degree of financial competence also can help to inform interpretations of the evidence regarding their financial performance.

This chapter also has provided an overview of the mental and physical disorders that can affect financial capability. There are only a very limited number of conditions for which incapability may be determined based solely on the presence and severity of the condition itself; examples include severe intellectual disability; significant autism; or advanced Alzheimer's disease, frontotemporal dementia, or dementia with Lewy bodies. Because of the variations in symptoms over time, the variable impact of disorders on the individuals affected, and the lack of correlation in many cases between the severity of one's clinical symptoms and one's functional limitations, assessment of individuals' financial capability will be required in the vast majority of cases.

REFERENCES

American Psychiatric Association. 2013. *The Diagnostic and Statistical Manual of Mental Disorders: DSM-5*. Washington, DC: American Psychiatric Association.

Appelbaum, P. S., and T. Grisso. 1988. Assessing patients' capacities to consent to treatment. *New England Journal of Medicine* 319(25):1635-1638.

Barrett, J. J., K. J. Hart, J. T. Schmerler, K. Willmarth, J. A. Carey, and S. Mohammed. 2009. Criterion validity of the financial skills subscale of the Direct Assessment of Functional Status Scale. *Psychiatry Research* 166(2-3):148-157.

Bechara, A., and E. M. Martin. 2004. Impaired decision making related to working memory deficits in individuals with substance addictions. *Neuropsychology* 18(1):152-162.

Bickel, W. K., A. L. Odum, and G. J. Madden. 1999. Impulsivity and cigarette smoking: Delay discounting in current, never, and ex-smokers. *Psychopharmacology* 146(4):447-454.

Birkenmaier, J., and Q. Fu. 2015. The association of alternative financial services usage and financial access: Evidence from the National Financial Capability Study. *Journal of Family and Economic Issues* 1-11.

Bisiacchi, P. S., M. Brandimonte, G. O. Einstein, and M. A. McDaniel. 1996. The neuropsychological approach in the study of prospective memory. *Prospective Memory: Theory and Applications* 219-237.

Black, A. C., and M. I. Rosen. 2011. A money management-based substance use treatment increases valuation of future rewards. *Addictive Behaviors* 36(1-2):125-128.

Borras, L., S. Mohr, M. Boucherie, S. Dupont-Willemin, F. Ferrero, and P. Huguelet. 2007. Patients with schizophrenia and their finances: How they spend their money. *Social Psychiatry and Psychiatric Epidemiology* 42(12):977-983.

Boyle, G. 2008. The Mental Capacity Act 2005: Promoting the citizenship of people with dementia? *Health & Social Care in the Community* 16(5):529-537.

Boyle, G. 2013. "She's usually quicker than the calculator": Financial management and decision-making in couples living with dementia. *Health & Social Care in the Community* 21(5):554-562.

Bradshaw, J., M. Saling, M. Hopwood, V. Anderson, and A. Brodtmann. 2004. Fluctuating cognition in dementia with Lewy bodies and Alzheimer's disease is qualitatively distinct. *Journal of Neurology, Neurosurgery, and Psychiatry* 75(3):382-387.

Brobeck, S. 2008. *Understanding the emergency savings needs of low-and moderate-income households: A survey-based analysis of impacts, causes, and remedies.* Washington, DC: Consumer Federation of America.

Buchanan, A. E., and D. W. Brock. 1989. *Deciding for others: The ethics of surrogate decision making.* Cambridge, UK: Cambridge University Press.

Capuano, A., and I. Ramsay. 2011. *What causes suboptimal financial behaviour? An exploration of financial literacy, social influences and behavioural economics.* University of Melbourne Legal Studies Research Paper No. 540. Melbourne, Australia: The University of Melbourne.

Carpenter-Song, E. 2012. Anthropological perspectives on money management: Considerations for the design and implementation of interventions for substance abuse. *The American Journal of Drug and Alcohol Abuse* 38(1):49-54.

Charland, L. C. 1998. Appreciation and emotion: Theoretical reflections on the MacArthur Treatment Competence Study. *Kennedy Institute of Ethics Journal* 8(4):359-376.

Charland, L. C. 2015. Decision-making capacity. In *Stanford encyclopedia of philosophy*, edited by E. N. Zalta. Stanford, CA: Stanford Center for the Study of Language and Information.

Claycomb, M., A. C. Black, C. Wilber, S. Brocke, C. Lazar, and M. I. Rosen. 2013. Financial victimization of adults with severe mental illness. *Psychiatric Services* 64(9):918-920.

Coffey, S. F., G. D. Gudleski, M. E. Saladin, and K. T. Brady. 2003. Impulsivity and rapid discounting of delayed hypothetical rewards in cocaine-dependent individuals. *Experimental and Clinical Psychopharmacology* 11(1):18-25.

Davidson, G., B. Kelly, G. Macdonald, M. Rizzo, L. Lombard, O. Abogunrin, V. Clift-Matthews, and A. Martin. 2015. Supported decision making: A review of the international literature. *International Journal of Law and Psychiatry* 38:61-67.

DiNicola, M., D. Tedeschi, M. Mazza, G. Martinotti, D. Harnic, V. Catalano, A. Bruschi, G. Pozzi, P. Bria, and L. Janiri. 2010. Behavioural addictions in bipolar disorder patients: Role of impulsivity and personality dimensions. *Journal of Affective Disorders* 125(1):82-88.

Drake, R. E., A. I. Alterman, and S. R. Rosenberg. 1993. Detection of substance use disorders in severely mentally ill persons. *Community Mental Health Journal* 29(2):175-192; discussion 193-194.

Drane, J. F. 1985. The many faces of competency. *Hastings Center Report* 15(2):17-21.

Dreer, L. E., M. J. DeVivo, T. A. Novack, and D. C. Marson. 2012. Financial capacity following traumatic brain injury: A six-month longitudinal study. *Rehabilitation Psychology* 57(1):5-12.

Duncan, A., and S. Bishop. 2013. Understanding the gaps between cognitive abilities and daily living skills in adolescents with autism spectrum disorders with average intelligence. *Autism* 9(1):64-72.

Eack, S. M., A. L. Bahork, S. A. McKnight, S. S. Hogarty, D. P. Greenwald, C. E. Newhill, M. L. Phillips, M. S. Keshavan, and N. J. Minshew. 2013. Commonalities in social and non-social cognitive impairments in adults with autism spectrum disorder and schizophrenia. *Schizophrenia Research* 148(1-3):24-28.

Earnst, K. S., V. G. Wadley, T. M. Aldridge, A. B. Steenwyk, A. E. Hammond, L. E. Harrell, and D. C. Marson. 2001. Loss of financial capacity in Alzheimer's disease: The role of working memory. *Aging, Neuropsychology, and Cognition* 8(2):109-119.

Elliott, R. 2003. Executive functions and their disorders. *British Medical Bulletin* 65:49-59.

Falicov, C. J. 2001. The cultural meanings of money the case of Latinos and Anglo-Americans. *American Behavioral Scientist* 45(2):313-328.

FDIC (Federal Deposit Insurance Corporation). 2014. *FDIC national survey of unbanked and underbanked households*. Washington, DC: FDIC.

Fisher, A. G., and L. A. Griswold. 2014. Performance skills: Implementing performance analyses to evaluate quality of occupational performance. In *Willard & Spackman's occupational therapy*, 12th ed., edited by B. B. Schell, G. Gillen, M. Scaffa, and E. Cohn. Philadelphia, PA: Lippincott Williams & Wilkins. Pp. 249-264.

Fiske, S. T., and S. E. Taylor. 2013. *Social cognition: From brains to culture*, 2nd ed. London, UK: Sage Publications Ltd.

Forgeot d'Arc, B. F., F. Ramus, A. Lefebvre, D. Brottier, T. Zalla, S. Moukawane, F. Amsellem, L. Letellier, H. Peyre, M. C. Mouren, M. Leboyer, and R. Delorme. 2014. Atypical social judgment and sensitivity to perceptual cues in autism spectrum disorders. *Journal of Autism and Developmental Disorders* [Epub ahead of print]. http://link.springer.com/article/10.1007%2Fs10803-014-2208-5 (accessed February 24, 2016).

Frank, J. B., and D. Degan. 1997. Conservatorship for the chronically mentally ill: Review and case series. *International Journal of Law and Psychiatry* 20(1):97-111.

Frith, C. D., and U. Frith. 2012. Mechanisms of social cognition. *Annual Review of Psychology* 63:287-313.

Gilloty, L., K. Kenworthy, L. Sirian, D. O. Black, and A. E. Wagner. 2002. Adaptive skills and executive function in autism spectrum disorders. *Neuropsychology* 8(4):241-248.

Goldfinger, S. M., R. K. Schutt, G. S. Tolomiczenko, L. Seidman, W. E. Penk, W. Turner, and B. Caplan. 1999. Housing placement and subsequent days homeless among formerly homeless adults with mental illness. *Psychiatric Services* 50(5):674-679.

Griffith, H. R., K. Belue, A. Sicola, S. Krzywanski, E. Zamrini, L. Harrell, and D. C. Marson. 2003. Impaired financial abilities in mild cognitive impairment: A direct assessment approach. *Neurology* 60(3):449-457.

Griffith, H. R., C. C. Stewart, L. E. Stoeckel, O. C. Okonkwo, J. A. Den Hollander, R. C. Martin, K. Belue, J. N. Copeland, L. E. Harrell, J. C. Brockington, D. G. Clark, and D. C. Marson. 2010. Magnetic resonance imaging volume of the angular gyri predicts financial skill deficits in people with amnestic mild cognitive impairment. *Journal of the American Geriatrics Society* 58(2):265-274.

Grisso, T. 2005. *Evaluating competencies: Forensic assessments and instruments*, 2nd ed., Vol. 16. New York: Springer Science & Business Media.

Grossman, L. S., J. K. Willer, N. S. Miller, J. G. Stovall, S. G. McRae, and S. Maxwell. 1997. Temporal patterns of veterans' psychiatric service utilization, disability payments, and cocaine use. *Journal of Psychoactive Drugs* 29(3):285-290.

Hernandez-Cardenache, R., L. Burguera, A. Acevedo, R. Curiel, and D. A. Loewenstein. 2014. Evaluating different aspects of prospective memory in amnestic and nonamnestic mild cognitive impairment. *ISRN Neurology* 2014:1-7.

Hilgert, M. A., J. M. Hogarth, and S. G. Beverly. 2003. Household financial management: The connection between knowledge and behavior. *Federal Reserve Bulletin* 89(7):309-322.

Hsu, J. W., and R. Willis. 2013. Dementia risk and financial decision making by older households: The impact of information. *Journal of Human Capital* 2013:45.

IOM (Institute of Medicine). 1991. *Disability in America: Toward a national agenda for prevention*. Washington, DC: National Academy Press.

IOM. 1997. *Enabling America: Assessing the role of rehabilitation science and engineering*. Washington, DC: National Academy Press.

IOM. 2007. *A 21st century system for evaluating veterans for disability benefits*. Washington, DC: The National Academies Press.

IOM. 2015. *Psychological testing in the service of disability determination*. Washington, DC: The National Academies Press.

Karantzoulis, S., A. K. Troyer, and J. B. Rich. 2009. Prospective memory in amnestic mild cognitive impairment. *Journal of the International Neuropsychological Society* 15(3):407-415.

Kazui, H., A. Matsuda, N. Hirono, E. Mori, N. Miyoshi, A. Ogino, H. Tokunaga, Y. Ikejiri, and M. Takeda. 2005. Everyday memory impairment of patients with mild cognitive impairment. *Dementia and Geriatric Cognitive Disorders* 19(5-6):331-337.

Kehiaian, S. E. 2012. *Factors and behaviors that influence financial literacy in US households*. Ph.D. dissertation, Nova Southeastern University.

Kim, S. Y. H., and P. S. Appelbaum. 2006. The capacity to appoint a proxy and the possibility of concurrent proxy directives. *Behavioral Sciences and the Law* 24(4):469-478.

Kim, S. Y. H., J. Karlawish, H. M. Kim, I. F. Wall, A. Bozoki, and P. S. Appelbaum. 2011. Preservation of the capacity to appoint a proxy decision maker: Implications for dementia research. *Archives of General Psychiatry* 68(2):214-220.

Kirby, K. N., and N. M. Petry. 2004. Heroin and cocaine abusers have higher discount rates for delayed rewards than alcoholics or non-drug-using controls. *Addiction* 99(4):461-471.

Kliegel, M., M. Martin, M. McDaniel, and G. O. Einstein. 2002. Complex prospective memory and executive control of working memory: A process model. *Psychological Test and Assessment Modeling* 44(2):303-318.

Knight, A. J., and D. C. Marson. 2012. The emerging neuroscience of financial capacity. *Generations* 36(2):46-52.

Lazar, C. M., A. C. Black, T. J. McMahon, R. A. Rosenheck, R. Ries, D. Ames, and M. I. Rosen. 2015a. All-data approach to assessing financial capability in people with psychiatric disabilities. *Psychological Assessment* [Epub ahead of print]. http://dx.doi.org/10.1037/pas0000179 (accessed February 24, 2016).

Lazar, C. M., A. C. Black, T. J. McMahon, K. O'Shea, and M. I. Rosen. 2015b. Ambiguity in determining financial capability of SSI and SSDI beneficiaries with psychiatric disabilities. *Psychiatric Services* 66(3):279-284.

Lee, D. R., J. P. Taylor, and A. J. Thomas. 2012. Assessment of cognitive fluctuation in dementia: A systematic review of the literature. *International Journal of Geriatric Psychiatry* 27(10):989-998.

Lichtenberg, P. A. 2015. Financial decision making in the midst of cognitive decline. Presentation to the Committee to Evaluate the Social Security Administration's Capability Determination Process for Adult Beneficiaries, June 24, Washington, DC.

Lipton, F. R., C. Siegel, A. Hannigan, J. Samuels, and S. Baker. 2000. Tenure in supportive housing for homeless persons with severe mental illness. *Psychiatric Services* 51(4):479-486.

Lusardi, A., and O. S. Mitchell. 2011. *Financial literacy around the world: An overview*. Working Paper 17107. Cambridge, MA: National Bureau of Economic Research.

Marks, L., D. C. Dollahite, and J. Dew. 2009. Enhancing cultural competence in financial counseling and planning: Understanding why families make religious contributions. *Journal of Financial Counseling and Planning* 20(2):14-26.

Marson, D. C. 2013. Clinical and ethical aspects of financial capacity in dementia: A commentary. *American Journal of Geriatric Psychiatry* 21(4):382-390.

Marson, D. C. 2015. Assessing financial capacity: A brief overview. Presentation to the Committee to Evaluate the Social Security Administration's Capability Determination Process for Adult Beneficiaries, April 21, Washington, DC.

Marson, D. C., S. M. Sawrie, S. Snyder, B. McInturff, T. Stalvey, A. Boothe, T. Aldridge, A. Chatterjee, and L. E. Harrell. 2000. Financial capacity instrument: Assessing financial capacity in patients with Alzheimer disease. *Archives of Neurology* 57(6):877-884.

Marson, D. C., R. Savage, and J. Phillips. 2006. Financial capacity in persons with schizophrenia and serious mental illness: Clinical and research ethics aspects. *Schizophrenia Bulletin* 32(1):81-91.

Martin, R. C., K. Triebel, L. E. Dreer, T. A. Novack, C. Turner, and D. C. Marson. 2012. Neurocognitive predictors of financial capacity in traumatic brain injury. *Journal of Head Trauma Rehabilitation* 27(6):E81-E90.

Matthews, N. L., C. J. Smith, E. Pollard, S. Ober-Reynolds, J. Kirwan, and A. Malligo. 2015. Adaptive functioning in autism spectrum disorder during the transition to adulthood. *Journal of Autism and Developmental Disorders* 45(8):2349-2360.

McDaniel, M. A., and G. O. Einstein. 2000. Strategic and automatic processes in prospective memory retrieval: A multi-process framework. *Applied Cognitive Psychology* 14(7):S127-S144.

Morgan-Cross, C. J., and Klawitter, M. 2011. *Alternative financial services use across income, race and ethnic groups*. University of Washington, Evans School of Public Affairs. http://d7stage.evans.uw.edu/sites/default/files/public/NWAF%20AFS%20review%20FINAL.pdf (accessed February 11, 2016).

Moye, J., and D. C. Marson. 2007. Assessment of decision-making capacity in older adults: An emerging area of practice and research. *Journals of Gerontology—Series B Psychological Sciences and Social Sciences* 62(1):P3-P11.

Moye, J., J. C. Armesto, and M. J. Karel. 2005. Evaluating capacity of older adults in rehabilitation settings: Conceptual models and clinical challenges. *Rehabilitation Psychology* 50(3):207-214.

Mullainathan, S., and E. Shafir. 2013. *Scarcity: Why having too little means so much*. New York: Time Books, Henry Holt & Company LLC.

Najt, P., J. Perez, M. Sanches, M. A. M. Peluso, D. Glahn, and J. C. Soares. 2007. Impulsivity and bipolar disorder. *European Neuropsychopharmacology* 17(5):313-320.

National Conference of Commissioners on Uniform State Laws. 1997. *Uniform Guardianship and Protective Proceedings Act (1997/1998)*. http://www.uniformlaws.org/shared/docs/guardianship%20and%20protective%20proceedings/UGPPA_2011_Final%20Act_2014sep9.pdf (accessed February 11, 2016).

Niekawa, N., Y. Sakuraba, H. Uto, Y. Kumazawa, and O. Matsuda. 2007. Relationship between financial competence and cognitive function in patients with schizophrenia. *Psychiatry and Clinical Neurosciences* 61(5):455-461.

North, C. S., D. E. Pollio, E. M. Smith, and E. L. Spitznagel. 1998. Correlates of early onset and chronicity of homelessness in a large urban homeless population. *Journal of Nervous and Mental Disease* 186(7):393-400.

OIDAP (Occupational Information Development Advisory Panel). 2009. *Mental cognitive subcommittee: Content model and classification recommendations*. https://www.ssa.gov/oidap/Documents/AppendixC.pdf (accessed February 11, 2016).

Okonkwo, O. C., V. G. Wadley, H. R. Griffith, K. Ball, and D. C. Marson. 2006. Cognitive correlates of financial abilities in mild cognitive impairment. *Journal of the American Geriatrics Society* 54(11):1745-1750.

Okonkwo, O. C., V. G. Wadley, H. R. Griffith, K. Belue, S. Lanza, E. Y. Zamrini, L. E. Harrell, J. C. Brockington, D. Clark, R. Raman, and D. C. Marson. 2008. Awareness of deficits in financial abilities in patients with mild cognitive impairment: Going beyond self-informant discrepancy. *American Journal of Geriatric Psychiatry* 16(8):650-659.

Olfson, M., D. Mechanic, S. Hansell, C. A. Boyer, and J. Walkup. 1999. Prediction of homelessness within three months of discharge among inpatients with schizophrenia. *Psychiatric Services* 50(5):667-673.

Palmer, H. M., and S. McDonald. 2000. The role of frontal and temporal lobe processes in prospective remembering. *Brain and Cognition* 44(1):103-107.

Payne, S. H., J. B. Yorgason, and J. P. Dew. 2014. Spending today or saving for tomorrow: The influence of family financial socialization on financial preparation for retirement. *Journal of Family and Economic Issues* 35(1):106-118.

Petry, N. M. 2001. Delay discounting of money and alcohol in actively using alcoholics, currently abstinent alcoholics, and controls. *Psychopharmacology* 154(3):243-250.

Pirogovsky, E., S. P. Woods, J. V. Filoteo, and P. E. Gilbert. 2012. Prospective memory deficits are associated with poorer everyday functioning in Parkinson's disease. *Journal of the International Neuropsychological Society* 18(6):986-995.

Prager, R. A. 2014. Determinants of the locations of alternative financial service providers. *Review of Industrial Organization* 45(1):21-38.

President's Commission for the Study of Ethical Problems in Medicine and Biomedical and Behavioral Research. 1982. *Making health care decisions*, Vol. 1. Washington, DC: President's Commission for the Study of Ethical Problems in Medicine and Biomedical and Behavioral Research.

Regier, D. A., M. E. Farmer, D. S. Rae, B. Z. Locke, S. J. Keith, L. L. Judd, and F. K. Goodwin. 1990. Comorbidity of mental disorders with alcohol and other drug abuse: Results from the Epidemiologic Catchment Area (ECA) Study. *Journal of the American Medical Association* 264(19):2511-2518.

Rosen, M. I., R. A. Rosenheck, A. L. Shaner, T. A. Eckman, G. R. Gamache, and C. W. Krebs. 2002. Substance abuse and the need for money management assistance among psychiatric inpatients. *Drug and Alcohol Dependence* 67(3):331-334.

Rosen, M. I., R. Rosenheck, and K. Ablondi. 2008. *ATM: A clinician manual to conduct money management with your clients*. http://www.behaviorchange.yale.edu/interventions/ATM-ManualFinal_tcm363-37151_tcm363-284-32.pdf (accessed January 30, 2016).

Rosen, M. I., B. J. Rounsaville, K. Ablondi, A. C. Black, and R. A. Rosenheck. 2010. Advisor-Teller Money Manager (ATM) therapy for substance use disorders. *Psychiatric Services* 61(7):707-713.

Roth, L. H., A. Meisel, and C. W. Lidz. 1977. Tests of competency to consent to treatment. *American Journal of Psychiatry* 134(3):279-284.

Sabatino, C. P., and S. L. Basinger. 2000. Competency: Reforming our legal fictions. *Journal of Mental Health and Aging* 6(2):119-144.

Sakuraba, Y., Y. Kumawzawa, and O. Matsuda. 2004. Development of the Financial Competency Assessment Tool (FCAT): A study of the reliability and validity of the FCAT. *Bulletin of Tokyo Gakugei University Section I Science Education* 55:131-139 (in Japanese).

Shafir, E. 2015 (unpublished). *Context & capability*. Princeton, NJ: Princeton University.

Shaner, A., T. A. Eckman, L. J. Roberts, J. N. Wilkins, D. E. Tucker, J. W. Tsuang, and J. Mintz. 1995. Disability income, cocaine use, and repeated hospitalization among schizophrenic cocaine abusers—a government-sponsored revolving door? *New England Journal of Medicine* 333(12):777-783.

Sherod, M. G., H. R. Griffith, J. Copeland, K. Belue, S. Krzywanski, E. Y. Zamrini, L. E. Harrell, D. G. Clark, J. C. Brockington, R. E. Powers, and D. C. Marson. 2009. Neurocognitive predictors of financial capacity across the dementia spectrum: Normal aging, mild cognitive impairment, and Alzheimer's disease. *Journal of the International Neuropsychological Society* 15(2):258-267.

Sherraden, M. S. 2013. Building blocks of financial capability. In *Financial education and capability: Research, education, policy, and practice*, edited by J. Birkenmaier, M. Sherraden, and J. Curley. New York: Oxford University Press. Pp. 3-43.

Shulman, K. I., I. M. Hull, S. DeKoven, S. Amodeo, B. J. Mainland, and N. Herrmann. 2015. Cognitive fluctuations and the lucid interval in dementia: Implications for testamentary capacity. *Journal of the American Academy of Psychiatry and the Law* 43(3):287-292.

Smith, L. E., M. J. Maenner, and M. M. Seltzer. 2012. Developmental trajectories in adolescents and adults with autism: The case of daily living skills. *Journal of the American Academy of Child and Adolescent Psychiatry* 51(6):622-631.

SSA (U.S. Social Security Administration). 1996. *SSR 96-3p: Policy interpretation ruling. Titles II and XVI: Considering allegations of pain and other symptoms in determining whether a medically determinable impairment is severe.* http://www.socialsecurity.gov/OP_Home/rulings/di/01/SSR96-03-di-01.html (accessed November 9, 2015).

SSA. 2015a. *DI 23001.005 Disability Determination Services (DDS) procedures for developing capability.* https://secure.ssa.gov/poms.nsf/lnx/0423001005 (accessed November 9, 2015).

SSA. 2015b. *GN 00502.010 Capability determination—overview.* https://secure.ssa.gov/poms.nsf/lnx/0200502010 (accessed August 4, 2015).

SSA. n.d.-a. *Compassionate allowances conditions.* https://www.ssa.gov/compassionateallowances/conditions.htm (accessed November 9, 2015).

SSA. n.d.-b. *Disability evaluation under Social Security—listing of impairments: Adult listings (Part A).* https://www.ssa.gov/disability/professionals/bluebook/AdultListings.htm (accessed November 9, 2015).

SSA. n.d.-c. *Disability evaluation under Social Security—Part III: Listing of impairments.* http://www.ssa.gov/disability/professionals/bluebook/listing-impairments.htm (accessed November 9, 2015).

SSA. n.d.-d. *Disability evaluation under Social Security—Part III: Listing of impairments: Adult listings (Part A)—section 12.00 mental disorders.* http://www.ssa.gov/disability/professionals/bluebook/12.00-MentalDisorders-Adult.htm (accessed November 9, 2015).

SSA. n.d.-e. *Disability evaluation under Social Security—Part III: Listing of impairments: Adult listings (Part A)—section 12.02 organic mental disorders.* https://www.ssa.gov/disability/professionals/bluebook/12.00-MentalDisorders-Adult.htm#12_02 (accessed November 9, 2015).

SSA. n.d.-f. *Disability evaluation under Social Security—Part III: Listing of impairments: Adult listings (Part A)—section 12.05 intellectual disability.* https://www.ssa.gov/disability/professionals/bluebook/12.00-MentalDisorders-Adult.htm#12_05 (accessed November 9, 2015).

Stoeckel, L. E., C. C. Stewart, H. R. Griffith, K. Triebel, O. C. Okonkwo, J. A. den Hollander, R. C. Martin, K. Belue, J. N. Copeland, L. E. Harrell, J. C. Brockington, D. G. Clark, and D. C. Marson. 2013. MRI volume of the medial frontal cortex predicts financial capacity in patients with mild Alzheimer's disease. *Brain Imaging and Behavior* 7(3):282-292.

Stoesz, D. 2014. The consolidation of the secondary financial services market. *Journal of Sociology and Social Welfare* 41(3):115-132.

Suto, W. M., I. C. Clare, A. J. Holland, and P. C. Watson. 2005a. Capacity to make financial decisions among people with mild intellectual disabilities. *Journal of Intellectual Disability Research* 49(Pt. 3):199-209.

Suto, W. M. I., I. C. H. Clare, A. J. Holland, and P. C. Watson. 2005b. The relationships among three factors affecting the financial decision-making abilities of adults with mild intellectual disabilities. *Journal of Intellectual Disability Research* 49(3):210-217.

Suto, W. M. I., I. C. H. Clare, A. J. Holland, and P. C. Watson. 2006. Understanding of basic financial concepts among adults with mild learning disabilities. *British Journal of Clinical Psychology* 45(2):261-266.

Tepper, A. M., and A. Elwork. 1984. Competence to consent to treatment as a psychological construct. *Law and Human Behavior* 8(3-4):205-223.

Triebel, K. L., R. Martin, H. R. Griffith, J. Marceaux, O. C. Okonkwo, L. Harrell, D. Clark, J. Brockington, A. Bartolucci, and D. C. Marson. 2009. Declining financial capacity in mild cognitive impairment: A 1-year longitudinal study. *Neurology* 73(12):928-934.

United Nations. 2007. *Convention on the rights of persons with disabilities and optional protocol.* http://www.un.org/disabilities/documents/convention/convoptprot-e.pdf (accessed December 16, 2015).

Williamson, C., O. Alcantar, J. Rothlind, D. Cahn-Weiner, B. L. Miller, and H. J. Rosen. 2010. Standardised measurement of self-awareness deficits in FTD and AD. *Journal of Neurology, Neurosurgery & Psychiatry* 81(2):140-145.

Willner, P., R. Bailey, R. Parry, and S. Dymond. 2010a. Evaluation of the ability of people with intellectual disabilities to "weigh up" information in two tests of financial reasoning. *Journal of Intellectual Disability Research* 54(4):380-391.

Willner, P., R. Bailey, R. Parry, and S. Dymond. 2010b. Performance in temporal discounting tasks by people with intellectual disabilities reveals difficulties in decision-making and impulse control. *American Journal on Intellectual and Developmental Disabilities* 115(2):157-171.

Willner, P., R. Bailey, S. Dymond, and R. Parry. 2011. Coins and costs: A simple and rapid assessment of basic financial knowledge. *Journal of Applied Research in Intellectual Disabilities* 24(3):285-289.

Wixon, B., and A. Strand, eds. 2013. *Identifying SSA's sequential disability determination steps using administrative data.* Research and statistics note no. 2013-01. https://socialsecurity.gov/policy/docs/rsnotes/rsn2013-01.html (accessed February 11, 2016).

Woods, S. P., J. E. Iudicello, L. M. Moran, C. L. Carey, M. S. Dawson, and I. Grant. 2008. HIV-associated prospective memory impairment increases risk of dependence in everyday functioning. *Neuropsychology* 22(1):110-117.

WHO (World Health Organization). 2001. *International Classification of Functioning, Disability and Health (ICF).* Geneva, Switzerland: WHO.

5

Methods and Measures for Assessing Financial Competence and Performance

Building on the conceptual framework of financial capability presented in the previous chapter, this chapter begins by providing an overview of the assessment of financial capability. This is followed by a description of the role and important characteristics of instruments for assessment of financial competence and performance, a review of instruments currently available, and a summary of their uses and limitations. Considerations and challenges entailed in financial capability assessment are then described.

OVERVIEW OF ASSESSMENT OF FINANCIAL CAPABILITY

The goal of financial capability assessment is to evaluate—as objectively as possible—an individual's abilities to manage or direct the management of his or her funds in a way that routinely meets the person's basic needs of food, shelter, and clothing. Assessment of financial capability involves the collection, integration, and interpretation of relevant information from a variety of sources. These sources of information may include

- interviews with the individual;
- behavioral observations of the individual;
- formal financial capability assessment instruments (e.g., structured interviews);
- records from physicians, psychologists, nurses, social workers, professional counselors, occupational therapists, rehabilitation counselors, and other health care professionals; and

- communication with and from knowledgeable third parties (e.g., family members, friends, nonlicensed professionals).

Assessments can be either direct or indirect. *Direct assessments* are those based on a sample of the individual's self-report or actual performance, whether it be in an office setting (i.e., interviews, observations, assessment instruments) or a real-life setting (observations). *Indirect assessment* refers to the collection of information from records or third parties (e.g., record review, interviews with individuals knowledgeable about the person's financial performance).

The setting in which an assessment takes place (e.g., a natural environment or a controlled setting such as a clinician's office) is important. As described in Chapters 1 and 4, the committee's conceptualization of financial capability distinguishes between *financial competence* (i.e., the financial knowledge and financial judgment one possesses, demonstrated in a controlled [e.g., office or clinical] setting) and *financial performance* (i.e., one's degree of success in handling financial demands in the context of the stresses, supports, contextual cues, resources, and opportunities in one's actual environment). Certain independent activities of daily living, such as shopping, managing one's finances, and arranging for transportation, are indicative of successful financial performance (Harvey et al., 2013; McKibbin et al., 2004). Direct assessment of a person's ability to meet the financial demands of his or her everyday environment, taking into account task complexity, compensatory abilities, and environmental supports, would be optimal. However, except for social workers, case workers, and other professionals who perform home assessments or otherwise interact with clients in their natural environment, professionals generally must rely on client self-report, collateral informants such as family members, or medical records from therapists or rehabilitation counselors in making judgments about financial performance. For this reason, formal instruments that provide valid and reliable information about an individual's financial capability could be useful in helping to inform the U.S. Social Security Administration's (SSA's) capability determinations.

INSTRUMENTS DESIGNED TO ASSESS FINANCIAL CAPABILITY

As part of its statement of task, SSA asked the committee to consider the use of assessment tools that could be employed in SSA's capability determination process. Many of the available instruments assess financial competence (financial knowledge and/or financial judgment) rather than real-world financial performance. The underlying assumption governing the use of these instruments is that the lack of the basic knowledge and skills required to identify and count currency or to employ basic arithmetic operations such as addition or subtraction will undermine a person's success in handling the financial demands of his or her everyday environment (Marson et al., 2000; Sherod et al., 2009). Similarly, if a person is unable to make financial choices that advance his or her best interests in response to hypothetical scenarios, the assumption is that the person also will be unable to do so in real life. Instruments used to assess financial knowledge and/or financial judgment collect information directly from the person's self-report; indirectly from collateral informants, such as family members or friends; or, increasingly, through direct observation of the ability of the person to perform calculations (Gerstenecker et al., 2015; Marson et al., 2000), work with actual currency (Marson et al., 2000), or make financial decisions in response to hypothetical scenarios (Marson et al., 2000).

Important Characteristics of Financial Capability Assessment Instruments

In its review of existing financial capability assessment instruments, the committee considered several important characteristics, including the instruments' reliability, validity, generalizability of performance, susceptibility to reporter biases, sensitivity and specificity, administration properties, and generalization to individuals with different disorders and of diverse ethnic and cultural backgrounds. Each of these characteristics is described in turn below.

Reliability

Reliability refers to the consistency of the results obtained from an assessment instrument. If a financial capability assessment instrument does not yield consistent results, the results are unreliable and cannot be interpreted meaningfully. Four types of reliability generally are assessed:

- *test-retest*—consistency of test scores over time (stability, temporal consistency);
- *interrater*—consistency of ratings or test scores across independent judges;
- *parallel- or alternative-forms*—consistency of scores across different forms of the test (stability and equivalence); and
- *internal consistency*—coherence of different items intended to measure the same thing within the test (homogeneity), a special case of which is *split-half reliability*, where scores on two halves of a single test are compared, and the result of this comparison can be converted into an index of reliability.

A number of factors can affect the reliability of a test's scores. These include the time elapsed between two administrations of the test, which affects test-retest and alternative-forms reliability; the scales of measurement applied (e.g., nominal versus interval); and similarity of content and expectations of subjects regarding different elements of the test, which affect alternative-forms and internal consistency (including split-half) reliability. Reliability also is affected by changes in subjects that occur over time and are introduced by physical ailments, emotional problems, or the subject's environment, as well as test-based factors such as poor test instructions, subjective scoring, and guessing. It is important to note that a test can generate reliable scores in one context and not in another, and that the inferences that can be drawn from different estimates of reliability are not interchangeable (Geisinger, 2013; IOM, 2015).

Validity

Validity is another important characteristic of assessment instruments. Historically, three primary types of validity have been recognized (Sattler, 2014; Sireci and Sukin, 2013):

- *construct validity*—the degree to which an instrument measures the theoretical concept it is designed to measure;
- *content validity*—the degree to which the instrument's content (typically reviewed by experts in the field) represents the targeted subject matter and supports use of the instrument for its intended purposes; and
- *criterion-related validity*—the degree to which the instrument's score correlates with other measurable, reliable, and relevant variables (i.e., criteria) thought to measure the same construct, which includes *concurrent validity* (high correlation with existing validated measures) and *predictive validity* (the extent to which an instrument's scores predict scores or outcomes on some criterion measure, such as future financial performance).

Generalizability of Performance

As previously noted, performance on a particular financial capability assessment instrument may differ in a laboratory or office setting and in the real world. For example, one might demonstrate the ability to count currency or make change for a purchase in a quiet clinical setting only to have difficulty in the real world at a busy supermarket. In such cases, performance on the instrument in a controlled setting cannot be generalized to performance in an individual's actual environment. If, as discussed in Chapter 4, financial performance is the most important component of financial capability for the purpose of determining the need for a representative payee, generalizability of performance is a critical property for a financial capability assessment instrument.

Susceptibility to Reporter Biases

Another characteristic of assessment instruments is susceptibility to reporter biases. To the extent that an instrument relies on information reported by the subject or a third-party informant, it is open to reporter biases. Persons can be poor reporters of their own financial capacities by virtue of having a memory or other cognitive impairment related to their condition (e.g., Alzheimer's dementia, schizophrenia), being unaware of their deficits related to brain injury (anosognosia), or minimizing their deficits for secondary gain (e.g., desiring autonomy in decision making). Third-party informants who know the person well can be helpful if they have ample opportunity to observe him or her in a variety of real-world situations, have the cognitive and psychological ability to make a proper assessment, and are motivated to convey accurate information. As discussed later in this chapter, however, not all informants are equally good reporters of financial performance, nor are all health care providers in a position to render accurate judgments about financial capability, given their lack of training in this area and their limited time and opportunities to assess financial capability in the individuals they see.

Sensitivity and Specificity

To be effective, any instrument used to determine deficits in financial capability needs to identify correctly a high percentage of persons who are truly impaired (sensitivity) while correctly excluding a high percentage of persons who are not impaired (specificity). For example, an instrument with a sensitivity of 85 percent and a specificity of 80 percent would correctly identify 85 percent of true cases of impairment but would miss 15 percent of true cases; and while 80 percent of nonimpaired cases would be correctly identified, 20 percent of cases would be falsely identified as impaired. It is important to note, however, that sensitivity and specificity are merely properties of assessment instruments. To determine the utility of an instrument, one needs to assess its true positive predictive value, which depends on its sensitivity and the actual base rate of impairment in the population, as well as its negative predictive value, which depends on its specificity and the population base rate.

Administration Properties

Ease and time of administration are important characteristics of any instrument used to determine financial knowledge, financial judgment, or financial performance. Instruments that take too long to administer may be impractical in clinical settings, where time is limited for practitioners and their staff. For some disorders, neuropsychological impairments that are characteristic of the disorder itself may mean that administration of even a relatively straightforward instrument may take a substantial amount of time. For example, the Financial Capacity Instrument (FCI) (Griffith et al., 2003; Marson et al., 2000) can take 40 to 50 minutes or longer to administer in a person with Alzheimer's disease. Other important administration properties include the nature and amount of training required to learn how to administer and score the test; whether the test relies on individual self-report or collateral information or is clinician rated; and how structured the instrument is (semistructured interviews require more training and judgment on the part of the interviewer relative to more structured instruments). Instruments whose administration requires trained individuals need to have clear scoring guidelines; the degree of structure of the scoring is another administration property.

Generalizability to Individuals with Different Disorders and of Diverse Ethnic and Cultural Backgrounds

Another characteristic that needs to be evaluated for each available instrument is external validity, or generalizability to individuals with different types of disorders and of diverse ethnic and cultural backgrounds. Given the diversity of current SSA beneficiaries with respect to cultural and language background as well as underlying medical, neurological, and neuropsychiatric conditions, it is important that any instruments used to assess financial capability be broadly generalizable.

Overview of Instruments Available for Assessing Financial Capability

The committee identified and reviewed eight instruments developed specifically to evaluate aspects of financial capability. Annex Table 5-1 at the end of this chapter summarizes information about each of these instruments, including its psychometric properties. Given the conceptual framework of financial capability described in Chapter 4, the committee examined each instrument in terms of the components of financial capability it is used to evaluate (as summarized in Table 5-1).[1] It should be noted that the committee is unaware of any instruments designed to assess individuals' ability to direct someone else to manage their funds.

[1] Because the instruments were developed independently of the conceptual framework proposed in Chapter 4, the committee inferred the components of the framework that may be assessed by the instruments from the type of data collected by each.

TABLE 5-1 Components of Financial Capability Measured by Assessment Instruments

Component of Financial Capability	Assessment Instruments
Financial Performance	Clinician Assessment of Financial Incapability (CAFI) (Black et al., 2014)
	Financial Incapability Structured Clinical Assessment done Longitudinally (FISCAL) (Lazar et al., 2015)
	Money Mismanagement Measure (MMM) (Conrad et al., 2006)
	Timeline Historical Review of Income and Financial Transactions (THRIFT) (Black et al., 2013)
Financial Knowledge	Financial Capacity Assessment Instrument (FCAI) (Kershaw and Webber, 2008)
	Financial Capacity Instrument (FCI) (Griffith et al., 2003; Marson et al., 2000)
	Financial Capacity Instrument-Short Form (FCI-SF) (Gerstenecker et al., 2015)
Financial Judgment	Assessment of Capacity for Everyday Decision-making (ACED) (Lai and Karlawish, 2007)
	CAFI
	FCAI
	FCI
	FISCAL
	MMM
	THRIFT

Assessment of Financial Performance

In contrast to financial knowledge and financial judgment, which can be measured in an office or clinical setting, financial performance represents the actual, real-world performance (or success) of an individual in handling financial demands in the context of the stresses, supports, contextual cues, and resources in his or her actual environment. Of the instruments reviewed by the committee, four appear to measure financial performance. The Financial Incapability Structured Clinical Assessment done Longitudinally (FISCAL) (Lazar et al., 2015) is focused on financial performance—particularly whether individuals have been spending their funds in a way that does not meet their basic needs or results in harm to them. The FISCAL incorporates information from the beneficiary's medical records, health care providers, and/or family members and information from a semistructured interview with the beneficiary (Rosen et al., 2015). The assessors reconcile any discrepancies among different sources of information, which helps offset the limitations of self-reported information (e.g., misrepresentation of one's circumstances or behavior). The FISCAL explicitly allows (but does not require) the use of contextual information to inform the determination of (what the instrument refers to as) "capability." The Clinician Assessment of Financial Incapability (CAFI) (Black et al., 2014) also appears to tap into financial performance, as it asks clinicians to rate how well the individual has been meeting his or her basic needs. Both instruments have showed good psychometric properties in relation to other assessment methods. The Money Mismanagement Measure (MMM) (Conrad et al., 2006), which was developed to help assess the effectiveness of representative payee systems, also relies on self-report to assess financial judgment and performance. Similarly, the Timeline Historical Review of Income and Financial Transactions (THRIFT) (Black et al., 2013) uses a timeline follow-back method to elicit information from individuals about their income, "in-kind" payments or exchanges (e.g., letting a friend stay in one's apartment in return for the friend's paying for food), expenditures, and debts over the past month, which can be used to evaluate the individuals' financial performance.

Assessment of Financial Knowledge

As described in Chapter 4, *financial knowledge* is possession of the declarative and procedural knowledge required to manage one's finances, including, for example, the concept of money, values of currency, making change, check writing, use of ATMs (automated teller machines), and online banking procedures. Three of the instruments listed in Table 5-1 can be used to assess financial knowledge, as measured by structured or semistructured questions that ask the individual to demonstrate knowledge or skills needed for managing finances or through observation of the individual carrying out financial or money-related tasks. Assessment of the kinds of knowledge measured by these instruments appears to require at least some level of clinical training, although a nonclinician arguably could be trained to administer them. Of the instruments reviewed, the Financial Capacity Instrument-Short Form (FCI-SF) (Gerstenecker et al., 2015) requires the least time to administer (approximately 15 minutes), as it is focused fairly narrowly on financial knowledge and calculations. The FCI is significantly longer (its administration to an individual with Alzheimer's disease, for example, can take 40 to 50 minutes), as it taps a broader range of financial skills, as well as financial judgment. The Financial Capacity Assessment Instrument (FCAI) also can be used to assess financial knowledge. The time required for its administration is not described (Kershaw and Webber, 2008).

Assessment of Financial Judgment

As discussed in Chapter 4, financial judgment is possession of the abilities needed to make financial decisions and choices that serve the individual's best interests. The FCI, which has been used primarily to assess financial knowledge in older adults with cognitive impairment, includes several items that can be used to assess financial judgment. These items are focused on the ability to detect mail and telephone fraud, schemes commonly used to exploit older adults. The FCAI (Kershaw and Webber, 2008) also purports to encompass financial judgment as one of the assessed domains; however, the committee found it difficult to determine whether this is actually the case. The FISCAL may implicitly measure financial judgment in that it provides a means of assessing whether the individual has been making decisions that serve his or her best interests, but it does not directly assess individuals' financial judgment, for example, in terms of their ability to make appropriate decisions on hypothetical scenarios. As indicated previously, it is more focused on actual performance. The MMM purports to measure financial judgment; as a self-report instrument, however, it is suited more for use as a screening tool than as a definitive measure of an individual's ability to make appropriate financial judgments. The THRIFT, through its use of the calendar timeline follow-back method, may tap into financial judgment (e.g., an individual may recall spending that was not in his or her best interests). However, it is difficult to determine how well this instrument can detect people's ability to protect their own best interests if they do not report any problems with their spending. The CAFI, designed as a clinician-rated instrument, assesses judgment through questions intended to determine whether an individual is at risk for financial victimization. Again, however, without direct observation of the individual, this instrument relies on the clinician's perspective and (in turn) on the individual's self-report.

The Assessment of Capacity for Everyday Decision-making (ACED) (Lai and Karlawish, 2007; Lai et al., 2008) was designed to help clinicians evaluate older adults' everyday decision-making capacity—particularly those with cognitive impairment whose ability to function independently at home may be in question. Issues commonly of concern in this population include the ability to manage one's finances. Therefore, the authors developed a specific version of the ACED's structured questionnaire to assess financial judgment—and possibly financial performance. Its format is modeled on the MacArthur tools developed by Appelbaum and Grisso to assess decision-making capacity for treatment (and later, for clinical research) (Lai et al., 2008). It has not been tested in individuals with serious mental illnesses such as schizophrenia.

General Functional Capacity Assessment Instruments with Financial Knowledge Subscales

A number of existing instruments are designed to assess functional capacity across a broad range of domains in adults with such conditions as schizophrenia, bipolar disorder, schizoaffective disorder, and major neurocognitive disorders (attributable to such conditions as Alzheimer's disease, Parkinson's dementia, diffuse Lewy body disease, frontotemporal dementia, head trauma, and vascular dementia)—conditions that may be present in Social Security beneficiaries being evaluated for capability. In reviewing the literature, the committee found a number of instruments designed to assess functional domains that may include or overlap with financial capability. Although these instruments were not designed specifically to assess financial performance and competence, several of them have validated financial knowledge subscales that can be used to assess such skills as identifying and counting currency, writing a check, and balancing a checkbook.

Two such instruments commonly used are the Independent Living Scales (ILS) (Loeb, 1996) and the Kohlman Evaluation of Living Skills (KELS) (Thomson, 1992). Both have established reliability and validity. The ILS is a standardized, individually administered assessment of adults' competence in independent activities of daily living, including managing money. The money management subscale assesses the individual's ability to count money, perform monetary calculations, pay bills, and take precautions with money. The items are both knowledge focused (e.g., inquiring about the cost of a loaf of bread) and performance focused (e.g., observing the person writing a check) within an office or clinical setting. Although originally developed for use in older adults, the ILS can be used with a variety of clinical populations. The money management subscale has good reliability (0.88), and its criterion and concurrent validity have been established. The KELS is a standardized, individually administered assessment of a person's possession of basic living skills, including money management. Originally developed for use in short-term psychiatric facilities, it can be used across populations. Specific items include making change, filling out bank forms, and paying bills.

More recently, the financial subscale of the UCSD Performance-based Skills Assessment (UPSA) (Patterson et al., 2001) and UPSA Brief (UPSA-B) (Mausbach et al., 2010, 2011) has been used to assess individuals with bipolar and schizoaffective disorders. This subscale enables direct assessment of such functional tasks as counting currency, making change for a purchase, and balancing a checkbook. Its advantage is that it has been shown to correspond to neurocognitive testing, has good discriminative validity, and has been used with different ethnic and cultural groups (Mausbach et al., 2010, 2011). Like the ILS and KELS, however, the UPSA subscale provides information only on financial competence as demonstrated in a test environment and does not capture real-world performance.

The functional tests of the financial subscale of the Everyday Functioning Battery (Heaton et al., 2004) are more advanced than the UPSA subscale. First developed to assess the financial skills of adults diagnosed with HIV infection, it was used more recently in the Valero study for persons with schizophrenia (Harvey et al., 2011). This instrument assesses higher-order functional skills such as preparing checks and bank deposits to pay bills, organizing specific payments, and setting aside specific amounts of money in a bank account.

The financial subscale of the information version of the Independent Living Skills Survey (ILSS) (Wallace et al., 2000) has been widely used among informants of persons with schizophrenia and other neuropsychiatric disorders. Questions focus on real-world performance as measured by the frequency of successfully performing acts requiring the assessed skills in the past 30 days; scores range from "never" to "always" (on a 0-4 point scale). In addition, the extent to which the individual performed the skilled acts without prompting is rated. Examples of the 10 items of the financial subscale include (1) paying bills for rent or utilities, (2) budgeting money and planning where money should be spent, (3) making a deposit or withdrawal from a bank, (4) cashing a paycheck or Supplemental Security Income (SSI) check, (5) purchasing essential items before luxury items, and (6) purchasing prescribed medication.

Because all of the above instruments were designed to assess functional capacity across a broad range of domains, none permits the comprehensive assessment of financial competence and performance enabled by instruments designed specifically for that purpose, despite having validated financial subscales. It should also be noted that, as with the latter instruments, none of these subscales directly taps the ability of individuals to manage their benefits directly, although the ILSS includes an item for informants to rate the degree to which a person contacted someone responsible for financial support and asked that individual relevant questions.

USES AND LIMITATIONS OF AVAILABLE ASSESSMENT INSTRUMENTS

The committee concludes that at present, because of their limitations, no single assessment instrument can be recommended for routine use with beneficiaries. Although the characteristics of the instruments vary, as a group they lack data demonstrating one or more of the following characteristics: construct and content validity for assessment of the ability to manage benefits to meet basic needs; ability to measure financial performance in a real-world (as opposed to office or clinical) setting; efficiency in administration;

ability to be administered reliably by a range of professionals; confirmation of reliability and validity when used by persons other than their developers; and validity for use with individuals with different disorders and of diverse ethnic and cultural backgrounds. Several of the instruments are also limited by reliance on self-report by the person being assessed.

Two of these limitations warrant emphasis. First, most of the available instruments were not developed specifically to evaluate the ability of SSA beneficiaries to manage their benefits to meet their basic needs. Hence, they may include items that relate to other financial functions and yield data that are not responsive to the question at hand. A particular risk in such situations is that beneficiaries will be deemed incapable based on assessment of tasks not directly related to the management of their benefits, or will have relevant impairments overlooked because they are not the focus of the instrument being used.

Second, most of the instruments were designed for use with individuals with specific disorders and therefore, without additional validation, cannot be generalized for use with individuals with different disorders or of diverse ethnic and cultural backgrounds. Given the diversity of conditions and paths that may lead to deficits in financial performance, it is reasonable to question whether a test developed for one condition is equally valid for another. For example, is a test developed for use in people with Alzheimer's disease or other neurocognitive conditions equally valid for persons with schizophrenia, bipolar disorder, major depression, or substance abuse? Moreover, many measures developed for U.S.-born, English-speaking individuals may not be relevant or appropriate for non-native English speakers or individuals of different cultural groups. As noted above, it is important that any instruments used to assess financial capability be broadly generalizable because current SSA beneficiaries represent a highly diverse population with respect to culture, language, and underlying conditions. The committee found little evidence that any of the available instruments has to date been sufficiently tested or validated in diverse populations.

When using these instruments, one must also take assessor bias into consideration. The assessment of financial judgment, in particular, can be affected by value judgments embedded in the design and scoring of the instrument being used. Bias can be reflected, for example, in the instrument's cut-off scores. Likewise, different perceptions of what is valuable can impact the assessment of financial judgment and performance. For instance, an individual may value setting aside a weekly allotment for a hair appointment even if it means having less money with which to buy food, while the assessor may deem weekly hair appointments excessive and unnecessary if they mean the person will not have enough food.

Although the committee currently cannot recommend any of the available instruments for routine use, ongoing study of existing instruments may in the future demonstrate their reliability and validity for assessments of beneficiaries' capability to manage or direct the management of their benefits. Even given the limitations of current instruments, however, the committee recognizes that individual clinicians or other assessors may find one or another instrument (particularly when validated for the population of which the person being assessed is a member) to be helpful in informing their judgments about individuals' capability.

CONSIDERATIONS AND CHALLENGES IN ASSESSMENT OF FINANCIAL COMPETENCE AND PERFORMANCE

Sources of Evidence

As noted at the beginning of this chapter, assessment of financial capability may be direct and/or indirect. The strength of direct assessment is that it captures the individual's actual ability in a given setting, but its primary limitation is that some capabilities (e.g., judgment, pursuit of one's best interests) cannot be assessed by direct observation. Direct assessment methods are subject to a number of other limitations as well. With respect to self-reported information, it is well established that people often are poor reporters of their true functional status and tend to overestimate their actual abilities (Bowie et al., 2007; Gould et al., 2015). Respondents' abilities to self-report accurately depend on a number of factors, including what they are reporting (the specific domain of functioning), whether the function is observable to others, and what health conditions the respondent may have that could affect reporting (i.e., conditions affecting insight or cognition). Direct observations also may be affected by observer bias or the setting in which the assessment takes place. For example, math tests in a formal, office setting may make some people anxious, which may result in underperformance in that setting.

Indirect assessment entails record review and/or collection of collateral information from third parties. Collateral reports from individuals knowledgeable about the beneficiary's financial performance in meeting his or her basic needs are especially useful when individuals, including those with significant psychiatric or cognitive disorders, cannot accurately provide direct information about their financial capability (e.g., they may provide inaccurate self-assessment or be unable to participate in direct assessment). Collateral informants (such as family members, neighbors, members of the clergy, and others who interact frequently with the beneficiary) can provide information based on their observations of the individual's financial knowledge, judgment, and performance in the real world. Recent work, however, has found that the quality of information provided by collateral informants varies (Kershaw and Webber, 2008; Sabbag et al., 2011). Some individuals may lack involved family members or friends who can provide reliable information about their financial performance. Some informants do not have the opportunity to observe financial performance (e.g., the person's making a purchase), while others spend insufficient time with the individual to assess his or her performance accurately. In addition, some collateral informants may under- or overestimate the individual's financial abilities. A relative might underestimate or underreport an individual's financial abilities in the hope of gaining access to the person's funds or overestimate the person's abilities so as not to alienate him or her.

Medical professionals often are asked to render judgments about financial capability (see, e.g., SSA's Form 787 in Appendix C). Medical professionals are trained diagnosticians, but as discussed in Chapter 4, diagnosis alone is seldom sufficient for making a judgment about financial capability. In addition, the majority of medical professionals lack specific training in how best to assess financial capability (Widera et al., 2011). Interviews with the individual during a clinical encounter may lead to inaccurate judgments about his or her financial capability. There is ample evidence that for many providers who do not know the client well, biased self-reports by beneficiaries may lead to inaccurate judgments (Loewenstein et al., 2001; Marson et al., 2006; Sabbag et al., 2011). Because diagnosis and medical evidence are less important than actual knowledge of a person's financial capabilities, medical professionals, including consultative examiners, who lack current information about the individual's real-world financial performance, who do not know the person well, or who lack access to good collateral informants or relevant records may not provide the most useful information to SSA about the person's financial capability.

Many other health and social service professionals, such as social workers, occupational therapists, caseworkers, and rehabilitation counselors, work regularly with clients and their families and therefore may have superior information about the client's financial knowledge and skills, financial judgment, and available environmental supports. Importantly, professionals who work more directly and regularly with clients can assess the consistency of their abilities to meet financial demands in the real world. Financial performance in real-world situations can best be captured by informants who have current knowledge of and experience with how the individual functions in his or her actual environment and have sufficient opportunities to observe the individual in that environment.

Social workers, for example, provide health, mental health, and substance abuse services in such positions as case manager, psychotherapist, rehabilitation counselor, medical social worker, behavioral analyst, and counselor. Social workers are employed in various service settings, such as primary care, specialty mental health care, community clinics, rehabilitation and recovery services, subsidized housing programs, and skilled nursing facilities that may give them access to direct observations of beneficiaries. Other relevantly trained professionals, such as nurses, physical therapists, occupational therapists, marriage and family counselors, and members of the clergy, often have direct knowledge of how individuals with whom they have regular contact function in their actual environment, as well as the supports they may have and the challenges they may face.

Given the potential difficulties with the use of medical evidence to inform determinations of financial capability, the committee endorses SSA's current requirement to consider what it calls "lay evidence" as part of its capability determination process. However, the committee notes that the strength of such evidence can vary depending on its source and that professionals with knowledge of individuals' performance may have insights beyond those attainable from nonprofessional informants (e.g., family members, neighbors). For this reason, it is important for SSA to distinguish between the weight given to "lay evidence" that comes from professionals (e.g., social workers, professional counselors, clergy) and that acquired from relatives, friends, landlords, and other untrained individuals.

Strength of Evidence

To help address the concerns outlined in the previous section, it is important that evidence of an individual's financial capability specify how well and for how long the informant has known the individual and the nature of their relationship.[2] It is also important to specify the extent to which (1) the informant's judgment is based on observed behavior; (2) the informant's judgment is based on the individual's self-report; (3) the informant's judgment is based on information from collateral informants, and the perceived quality of these informants; and (4) in the case of professionals, the judgment is based on the individual's medical record and the assessments of other health care professionals (including other physicians, psychologists, social workers, and nurses). Such specification of the basis for the evidence provided will allow for greater understanding of the quality of the evidence as support for a judgment regarding financial capability.

In addition, because most informants, including professionals, are not trained specifically in assessment of financial competence and performance, they would benefit from robust direction as to the type of information that is helpful in making a determination of financial capability. Providing such detailed guidance to professional and lay informants could be expected to improve the strength and quality of the evidence they provide. SSA recognizes that a face-to-face interview with the beneficiary is valuable for

[2] This would include, to the extent possible, the beneficiary's perspective on the relationship as well as the informant's.

determining capability and currently provides field office employees with sample questions to help guide them through the areas they may want to explore in an assessment of the beneficiary's capability (see Box 2-2 in Chapter 2). This same type of guidance would be helpful not just for SSA employees but for anyone being asked to provide information about an individual's financial performance. The FISCAL provides another source of questions that could be used to guide informants in acquiring and providing information about financial performance.

Evidence of financial competence may be needed to inform capability determinations when evidence of a beneficiary's real-world financial performance is very limited or unavailable, either because the person has had no funds to manage recently or because no reliable informant with such knowledge can be identified. Evidence of financial competence also could help to corroborate, refute, or explain evidence acquired of beneficiaries' financial performance. As with evidence of financial performance, detailed guidance and sample questions (see Box 5-1), with requests that the basis for informants' answers be specified, would assist informants in providing relevant information about beneficiaries' financial competence (knowledge and judgment).

The Need for Periodic Reassessment

An additional, important consideration emerged from the committee's review of methods and measures for assessing financial capability. As discussed in Chapter 4, many psychiatric and cognitive conditions are

BOX 5-1
Sample Questions About Financial Competence

Does the beneficiary have

1. Good general knowledge about what is happening to his or her money and investments?
2. Sufficient understanding of the concept of time, in order to pay bills promptly?
3. Sufficient memory to keep track of financial transactions and decisions?
4. Sufficient math and other skills to balance accounts and pay bills?
5. Significant impairment of judgment due to altered cognitive function?

SOURCE: Adapted from Service Canada's Certificate of Incapability (included in Appendix C).

characterized by progressive or fluctuating changes over time in the presence, severity, and nature of symptoms. Such changes make it difficult to assess capability as a static trait. (See Chapter 4 for a detailed discussion of this issue.) Without some mechanism for periodic reassessment, therefore, beneficiaries with fluctuating, deteriorating, or improving financial capability are more likely to be misclassified relative to those with more stable conditions. One possible approach to addressing this issue would be to incorporate reassessments of financial capability into the current process for continuing disability reviews (CDRs). For disability beneficiaries, SSA procedures call for periodic CDRs. Yet while CDRs provide a prime opportunity for capability (re)assessments, their purpose is to identify any changes (improvements) in the medical basis for beneficiaries' disability award. Thus, even if the CDRs were to occur on schedule, they would not fully serve the purpose of reassessment of financial capability.[3] SSA could apply the same principle used in the CDR process to develop an analogous process for recognizing and responding to changes in capability over time. Reassessments initially could be targeted toward (1) beneficiaries who had been determined to be incapable but who might improve over time as their condition or environmental supports changed; and (2) beneficiaries who, although capable, were at risk for becoming incapable as their condition progressed or their environment changed. As screening criteria or other systematic methods for identifying people at high risk for financial incapability were developed, they might be used to broaden the target population for periodic reassessment.

In addition, beneficiaries, family members, representative payees, and professionals who were likely to come into contact with beneficiaries could be alerted systematically to notify SSA if they believed that beneficiaries' capability had changed so as to warrant redetermination. SSA might also implement a process to survey payees and/or beneficiaries periodically, similar to that of the U.S. Office of Personnel Management, integrating screening questions that could trigger the need to further investigate the beneficiary's financial capability.

---

[3] For example, there are beneficiaries whose condition precludes their ability for substantial gainful activity but does not (yet) affect their financial competence or performance. When such a condition invariably will worsen, a CDR is required only every 5-7 years because the individual is not expected to regain the ability to work. As some of the conditions worsen, however, they may affect the individual's financial capability. Such cases are among those that are important for SSA to reevaluate.

SUMMARY

The chapter has provided a general overview of the uses and limitations of direct and indirect methods for assessing financial competence and financial performance. Of particular note are concerns about the reliability of self-reported information (e.g., due to an individual's lack of awareness of his or her impairment or deliberate efforts to conceal it) and of information about individuals' financial performance that is provided by third-party informants. Some informants lack the opportunity to observe financial performance, while others spend insufficient time with the individual to assess his or her performance accurately. Informants also may under- or overestimate the individual's financial abilities for a variety of reasons. In addition, most informants, including medical and nonmedical professionals, are not trained specifically in the assessment of financial performance and would benefit from robust direction as to the type of performance information that is helpful to SSA in making a determination of financial capability.

In principle, assessment instruments could be helpful to medical and other professionals in gathering evidence of beneficiaries' financial performance. However, half of the instruments identified by the committee are designed to assess financial competence in an office or clinical setting. Although four of the instruments appear to measure financial performance in a real-world setting, most rely primarily on self-reported behavior. While some of these instruments show good psychometric properties in relation to other assessment methods, sufficient data on reliability and validity across populations are not yet available to warrant recommending their routine use.

Although the committee currently cannot recommend any of the available instruments for routine use, ongoing study of existing instruments may in the future demonstrate their reliability and validity for assessment of beneficiaries' capability to manage or direct the management of their benefits. Even given the limitations of current instruments, however, the committee recognizes that individual clinicians or other assessors may find one or another instrument (particularly when validated for the population of which the person being assessed is a member) to be helpful in informing their judgments about individuals' capability.

REFERENCES

Black, A. C., K. L. Serowik, K. M. Ablondi, and M. I. Rosen. 2013. Timeline historical review of income and financial transactions: A reliable assessment of personal finances. *The Journal of Nervous and Mental Disease* 201(1):56-59.

Black, A. C., T. J. McMahon, R. A. Rosenheck, S. A. Ball, R. K. Ries, D. Ames, and M. I. Rosen. 2014. Development of the Clinician Assessment of Financial Incapability (CAFI). *Psychiatry Research* 215(3):784-789.

Bowie, C. R., E. W. Twamley, H. Anderson, B. Halpern, T. L. Patterson, and P. D. Harvey. 2007. Self-assessment of functional status in schizophrenia. *Journal of Psychiatric Research* 41(12):1012-1018.

Conrad, K. J., M. D. Matters, D. J. Luchins, P. Hanrahan, D. L. Quasius, and G. Lutz. 2006. Development of a money mismanagement measure and cross-validation due to suspected range restriction. *Journal of Applied Measurement* 7(2):206-224.

Geisinger, K. F. 2013. Reliability. In *APA handbook of testing and assessment in psychology*, Vol. 1, edited by K. F. Geisinger, B. A. Bracken, J. F. Carlson, J. C. Hansen, N. R. Kuncel, S. P. Reise, and M. C. Rodriguez. Washington, DC: American Psychological Association. Pp. 21-42.

Gerstenecker, A., A. Eakin, K. Triebel, R. Martin, D. Swenson-Dravis, R. C. Petersen, and D. Marson. 2015. Age and education corrected older adult normative data for a short form version of the financial capacity instrument. *Psychological Assessment* [Epub ahead of print].

Gould, F., L. S. McGuire, D. Durand, S. Sabbag, C. Larrauri, T. L. Patterson, E. W. Twamley, and P. D. Harvey. 2015. Self-assessment in schizophrenia: Accuracy of evaluation of cognition and everyday functioning. *Neuropsychology* 29(5):675-682.

Griffith, H. R., K. Belue, A. Sicola, S. Krzywanski, E. Zamrini, L. Harrell, and D. C. Marson. 2003. Impaired financial abilities in mild cognitive impairment: A direct assessment approach. *Neurology* 60(3):449-457.

Harvey, P. D., T. Raykov, E. W. Twamley, L. Vella, R. K. Heaton, and T. L. Patterson. 2011. Validating the measurement of real-world functional outcomes: Phase I results of the VALERO study. *The American Journal of Psychiatry* 168(11):1195-1201.

Harvey, P. D., L. Stone, D. Lowenstein, S. J. Czaja, R. K. Heaton, E. W. Twamley, and T. L. Patterson. 2013. The convergence between self-reports and observer ratings of financial skills and direct assessment of financial capabilities in patients with schizophrenia: More detail is not always better. *Schizophrenia Research* 147(1):86-90.

Heaton, R. K., T. D. Marcotte, M. Rivera Mindt, J. Sadek, D. J. Moore, H. Bentley, J. A. McCutchan, C. Reicks, and I. Grant. 2004. The impact of HIV-associated neuropsychological impairment on everyday functioning. *Journal of the International Neuropsychological Society* 10(3):317-331.

IOM (Institute of Medicine). 2015. *Psychological testing in the service of disability determination*. Washington, DC: The National Academies Press.

Kershaw, M. M., and L. S. Webber. 2008. Assessment of financial competence. *Psychiatry, Psychology and Law* 15(1):40-55.

Lai, J. M., and J. Karlawish. 2007. Assessing the capacity to make everyday decisions: A guide for clinicians and an agenda for future research. *The American Journal of Geriatric Psychiatry* 15(2):101-111.

Lai, J. M., T. M. Gill, L. M. Cooney, E. H. Bradley, K. A. Hawkins, and J. H. Karlawish. 2008. Everyday decision-making ability in older persons with cognitive impairment. *The American Journal of Geriatric Psychiatry* 16(8):693-696.

Lazar, C. M., A. C. Black, T. J. McMahon, R. A. Rosenheck, R. Ries, D. Ames, and M. I. Rosen. 2015. All-data approach to assessing financial capability in people with psychiatric disabilities. *Psychological Assessment* [Epub ahead of print].

Loeb, P. 1996. *Independent living scales*. San Antonio, TX: Psychological Corporation.

Loewenstein, D. A., S. Argüelles, M. Bravo, R. Q. Freeman, T. Argüelles, A. Acevedo, and C. Eisdorfer. 2001. Caregivers' judgments of the functional abilities of the Alzheimer's disease patient: A comparison of proxy reports and objective measures. *The Journals of Gerontology. Series B, Psychological Sciences and Social Sciences* 56(2):78-84.

Marson, D. C., S. M. Sawrie, S. Snyder, B. McInturff, T. Stalvey, A. Boothe, T. Aldridge, A. Chatterjee, and L. E. Harrell. 2000. Assessing financial capacity in patients with Alzheimer disease: A conceptual model and prototype instrument. *Archives of Neurology* 57(6):877-884.

Marson, D. C., R. Savage, and J. Phillips. 2006. Financial capacity in persons with schizophrenia and serious mental illness: Clinical and research ethics aspects. *Schizophrenia Bulletin* 32(1):81-91.

Martin, R. C., K. Triebel, R. E. Kennedy, A. P. Nicholas, R. L. Watts, N. Stover, M. Brandon, and D. C. Marson. 2013. Impaired financial abilities in Parkinson's disease patients with mild cognitive impairment and dementia. *Parkinsonism & Related Disorders* 19(11):986-990.

Mausbach, B. T., P. D. Harvey, A. E. Pulver, C. A. Depp, P. S. Wolyniec, M. H. Thornquist, J. R. Luke, J. A. McGrath, C. R. Bowie, and T. L. Patterson. 2010. Relationship of the Brief UCSD Performance-based Skills Assessment (UPSA-B) to multiple indicators of functioning in people with schizophrenia and bipolar disorder. *Bipolar Disorders* 12(1):45-55.

Mausbach, B. T., C. A. Depp, C. R. Bowie, P. D. Harvey, J. A. McGrath, M. H. Thronquist, J. R. Luke, P. S. Wolyniec, A. E. Pulver, and T. L. Patterson. 2011. Sensitivity and specificity of the UCSD Performance-based Skills Assessment (UPSA-B) for identifying functional milestones in schizophrenia. *Schizophrenia Research* 132(2-3):165-170.

McKibbin, C. L., J. S. Brekke, D. Sires, D. V. Jeste, and T. L. Patterson. 2004. Direct assessment of functional abilities: Relevance to persons with schizophrenia. *Schizophrenia Research* 72(1):53-67.

Patterson, T. L., S. Goldman, C. L. McKibbin, T. Hughs, and D. V. Jeste. 2001. UCSD Performance-Based Skills Assessment: Development of a new measure of everyday functioning for severely mentally ill adults. *Schizophrenia Bulletin* 27(2):235-245.

Rosen, M. I., A. C. Black, C. M. Lazar, R. A. Rosenheck, T. J. McMahon, and B. J. Rounsaville, in consultation with K. J. Conrad, R. Ries, and D. Ames. 2015. *Financial Incapability Structured Clinical Assessment done Longitudinally (F.I.S.C.A.L)* (Version 4/28/2015). New Haven, CT: Yale School of Medicine.

Sabbag, S., E. M. Twamley, L. Vella, R. K. Heaton, T. L. Patterson, and P. D. Harvey. 2011. Assessing everyday functioning in schizophrenia: Not all informants seem equally informative. *Schizophrenia Research* 131(1-3):250-255.

Sattler, J. M. 2014. *Foundations of behavioral, social, and clinical assessment of children*, 6th ed. La Mesa, CA: Jerome M. Sattler, Publisher, Inc.

Sherod, M. G., H. R. Griffith, J. Copeland, K. Belue, S. Krzywanski, E. Y. Zamrini, L. E. Harrell, D. G. Clark, J. C. Brockington, R. E. Powers, and D. C. Marson. 2009. Neurocognitive predictors of financial capacity across the dementia spectrum: Normal aging, mild cognitive impairment, and Alzheimer's disease. *Journal of the International Neuropsychological Society* 15(2):258-267.

Sireci, S. G., and T. Sukin. 2013. Test validity. In *APA handbook of testing and assessment in psychology*, Vol. 1, edited by K. F. Geisinger, B. A. Bracken, J. F. Carlson, J. C. Hansen, N. R. Kuncel, S. P. Reise, and M. C. Rodriguez. Washington, DC: APA. Pp. 61-84.

Thomson, L. K. 1992. *The Kohlman evaluation of living skills*, 3rd ed. Rockville, MD: American Occupational Therapy Association.

Wallace, C. J., R. P. Liberman, R. Tauber, and J. Wallace. 2000. The Independent Living Skills Survey: A comprehensive measure of the community functioning of severely and persistently mentally ill individuals. *Schizophrenia Bulletin* 26(3):631-658.

Widera, E., V. Steenpass, D. Marson, and R. Sudore. 2011. Finances in the older patient with cognitive impairment: "He didn't want me to take over." *Journal of the American Medical Association* 305(7):698-706.

ANNEX TABLE 5-1 Characteristics of Common Instruments for Assessing Financial Capability

Instrument (authors, year)	Domains/Items[a]	Component of Financial Capability Measured[b]	Administration Properties
Financial Incapability Structured Clinical Assessment done Longitudinally (FISCAL) (Lazar et al., 2015)	4 global criteria for financial incapability, scored using algorithm to yield dichotomous incapability determination: (A1) basic needs not met AND (A2) funds needed for basic needs were spent on something else; (B) substantial funds spent on something that harmed the client; (C1) past misspending (not meeting basic needs) likely to continue; (C2) past misspending (on harmful things) likely to continue Optional: contextual factors could be used to inform determination after algorithm yielded results	Financial performance; financial judgment	Clinician rated
Financial Capacity Instrument (FCI) (Griffith et al., 2003; Marson et al., 2000)	9 domains (activities), 18 tasks, 2 total scores (Marson et al., 2000: 6 domains, 14 tasks)	Financial knowledge; financial judgment	Training required to administer; 1 of the 9 domains requires collateral report Can take 40-50 minutes to administer to someone with Alzheimer's disease (AD)

Populations Studied	Psychometric Properties	Notes
118 adults (18-65 years; mean 46, standard deviation [SD] 10.5); ethnically diverse Inclusion criteria: inpatients in psychiatric unit or in intensive outpatient program; current or past *Diagnostic and Statistical Manual of Mental Disorders, Fourth Edition* (DSM-IV) substance use diagnosis; receiving ≥ $600 (Supplemental Security Income [SSI] or Social Security Disability Insurance [SSDI])/ month; no rep. payee or conservator	Face validity (expert reviewed) Interrater reliability: kappa = 0.77 ("very good") Construct validity: convergent validity with measure of money mismanagement (r = 0.46); discriminant validity with measure of depression (Beck Depression Inventory-II [BDI-II]; r = 0.24) Weak association with homelessness	Algorithm: A OR B met AND C met; optional use of contextual factors to inform determination; contextual factors invoked for 5 percent of cases (for disorganized behavior and impaired judgment) Higher agreement among raters when raters more certain of accuracy of their determinations Demographic characteristics did not differ between capable and incapable individuals
AD, mild cognitive impairment (MCI), Parkinson's disease (Martin et al., 2013), healthy older adults (as comparison groups)	In Marson et al. (2000) study, good reliability in each of the 6 reliability domains	Developed to assess financial decline in AD and related dementias; used primarily in research; limited clinical utility People with MCI (amnestic type) demonstrate significant impairments compared (in some but not all domains) with controls matched for age, sex, education, socioeconomic status (SES), and race; worse performance by MCI patients on practical application of concepts than on understanding of financial concepts

continued

ANNEX TABLE 5-1 Continued

Instrument (authors, year)	Domains/Items[a]	Component of Financial Capability Measured[b]	Administration Properties
Financial Capacity Instrument-Short Form (FCI-SF) (Gerstenecker et al., 2015)	5 domains assessed: coin/currency knowledge, financial conceptual knowledge and problem solving, understanding/using a checkbook, and understanding/using a bank statement Yields 5 scores (Mental Calculation, Financial Conceptual Knowledge, Single Checkbook/Register Task, Complex Checkbook/Register Task, and Using Bank Statement) Total score (range of 0-74); higher scores indicate better financial skills Also time-to-completion scores on a number of specific tasks and composite time scores	Financial knowledge	37 items, 15 minutes
Financial Capacity Assessment Instrument (FCAI) (Kershaw and Webber, 2008)	6 domain subscales, one total score Subscales: everyday financial abilities, financial judgment, estate management, cognitive functioning related to financial tasks, debt management, support resources	Financial knowledge; financial judgment	38 items (original had 41 items; 3 removed) Structured interview format; "objective scoring guidelines"

Populations Studied	Psychometric Properties	Notes
Cognitively normal, community-dwelling older adults (n = 1,344); ages 70-96		Developed from longer FCI; normative data available from original study (Gerstenecker et al., 2015); however, sample predominantly white Age significantly associated with performance scores (total and 4/5 domains) Education significantly associated with performance scores (total and all performance subtests)
Adults (n = 178, ages 18-91, mean 53) with cognitive impairment (defined by authors) due to acquired brain injury (n = 36), schizophrenia (n = 29), intellectual disability (n = 32), dementia (n = 22), and healthy controls (n = 59)	Internal consistency (Cronbach's alpha for subscales ranged from 0.54 to 0.91) Construct validity (positive correlations with other measures of financial competence) Interrater reliability; average 89 percent agreement (kappa = 0.86) Test-retest reliability high for 4/6 subscales and total score	People with a legally appointed administrator performed worse on all dimensions of FCAI compared with people without a legally appointed administrator

continued

ANNEX TABLE 5-1 Continued

Instrument (authors, year)	Domains/Items[a]	Component of Financial Capability Measured[b]	Administration Properties
Money Mismanagement Measure (MMM) (Conrad et al., 2006)	Questions re difficulties meeting basic needs, budgeting, paying bills, and keeping track of funds over past month; assesses financial situation	Financial judgment; possibly financial performance	28 items; self-reported
Timeline Historical Review of Income and Financial Transactions (THRIFT) (Black et al., 2013)	Uses calendar (timeline follow-back method) re past-month income, transactions, expenses, debt, and account balances	Financial judgment; financial performance	Semistructured interview
Clinician Assessment of Financial Incapability (CAFI) (Black et al., 2014)	Assesses spending, bill paying, management of funds, psychiatric symptoms, and ability to avoid financial victimization	Financial judgment; financial performance	32 items; structured questionnaire; clinician rated
Assessment of Capacity for Everyday Decision-making (ACED) (Lai and Karlawish, 2007; Lai et al., 2008)	Designed to assess capacity for "everyday" decisions (e.g., medication management); can be tailored to assess financial management	Financial judgment (understanding, appreciation, reasoning, expression of a choice)	Structured questionnaire consisting of 7 items, each scored 0, 1, or 2 Clinician rated and judged 15-20 minutes

[a] The "domains" listed in this column refer to those described by the authors, as opposed to the components of capability listed in the next column as determined by the committee.

[b] The components of financial capability measured by each instrument are listed here. These are based on the committee's judgment of which components are actually measured by an instrument, according to the committee's consensus definitions of financial capability, financial competence, financial knowledge, financial judgment, and financial performance (see Chapter 4).

Populations Studied	Psychometric Properties	Notes
Two samples of people with serious mental illness (SMI): (1) (n = 186, mean age 43); (2) (n = 184, mean age 46)	Rasch person reliability = 0.85 (in untreated sample; lower Rasch of 0.72 in original sample due to restriction of range) Good construct validity (expected correlations with other measures)	Screening assessment of money mismanagement for people with SMI Specifically developed with representative payee system in mind
People with SMI (n = 28)	1-week test-retest reliability: r = 0.77 (income); r = 0.91 (expenses); r = 0.99 (debt)	Available at www.behaviorchange.yale.edu
Patient-beneficiaries (n = 134) Mental health clinicians (n = 78), identified by patients as people who "could best answer questions about them for past 6 months"	Correctly classified 73 percent of cases in combination with SSA method (when compared with method described in FISCAL) Factor analysis supported expert-identified conceptual groupings of four subscales	Intended for use by treating clinician Available at www.behaviorchange.yale.edu
Patients with very mild to moderate cognitive impairment (n = 39); cognitively intact caregivers (n = 13)	Cronbach's alpha > 0.84 for each of 3 abilities assessed Moderate to strong correlation with MacArthur Competence Assessment Tool-Treatment (MacCAT-T); moderate correlations with measures of executive functioning	Designed for assessment of everyday decision-making capacity in older adults, particularly those with cognitive disorders Instrument and manual available from Jason Karlawish (jason.karlawish@uphs.upenn.edu).

6

Conclusions and Recommendations

The committee's conclusions and recommendations fall within the areas of (1) evidence for determining financial capability, (2) systematic identification of adult U.S. Social Security Administration (SSA) beneficiaries at risk for financial incapability, (3) responding to changes in capability over time, and (4) innovation and evaluation.

EVIDENCE FOR DETERMINING FINANCIAL CAPABILITY

The committee formulated the following conclusions and recommendation pertaining to determinations of financial capability for adult SSA beneficiaries.

- Because of the variations in symptoms over time, the variable impact of disorders on the individuals affected, and the lack of correlation in many cases between the severity of one's clinical symptoms and one's functional limitations, the number of conditions for which incapability may be determined solely on the presence and severity of the condition itself is very limited. Examples include severe intellectual disability; significant autism; or advanced Alzheimer's disease, frontotemporal dementia, or dementia with Lewy bodies.
- The committee distinguishes between financial competence (i.e., the financial knowledge and judgment one possesses) and financial performance (i.e., the degree of success in handling financial demands in the real world). Evidence of beneficiaries' real-world financial

performance in meeting their basic needs is the best indicator of financial capability, taking into account the nature of the beneficiaries' circumstances, including environmental barriers and supports.

Financial Performance

- Successful financial performance reflects, at a minimum, sufficient financial competence to implement financial decisions in the real world, that is, the presence of sufficient cognitive, perceptual, affective, communicative, and interpersonal abilities to manage or direct others to manage one's benefits.
- Supports and stressors in individuals' environments can enhance or diminish their (real-world) financial performance. Thus, one may be financially competent (i.e., possess and demonstrate financial knowledge and judgment) in an office or clinical setting but may not exercise one's financial knowledge, skills, and judgment in a real-life setting sufficiently to meet one's basic needs (food, shelter, clothing). Conversely, an individual may fail to demonstrate financial knowledge or judgment in a clinical setting but perform capably with the assistance of support systems in his or her environment.
- SSA's requirement for "lay" (i.e., nonmedical and nonlegal) evidence of beneficiaries' financial performance in making capability determinations is consistent with the committee's conclusion that evidence of real-world financial performance is the most reliable basis for making such determinations. Field officers are one source of lay evidence, particularly if they have had direct contact with beneficiaries. Other sources include professionals and laypeople who can provide nonmedical information relevant to beneficiaries' ability to manage or direct the management of their funds. However, the reliability of third-party informants varies. Some informants lack the opportunity to observe financial performance, while others spend insufficient time with the individual to assess his or her performance accurately. Some informants may have impaired judgment themselves, or may have an incentive to under- or overestimate the individual's financial abilities.
- Because many informants, including medical and nonmedical professionals, are not trained specifically in the assessment of financial performance, they would benefit from detailed direction as to the type of performance information that is helpful to SSA in making a determination of financial capability.
- SSA currently provides little formal guidance to medical professionals and no formal guidance to other informants on the type of

information on which an opinion regarding capability should be based or the type of information that would be helpful to SSA.

- In principle, assessment instruments could be helpful to medical and other professionals in gathering evidence of beneficiaries' financial performance. However, many of the instruments identified by the committee are designed to assess financial competence in an office or clinical setting. Some of the instruments appear to measure financial performance in a real-world setting, but most of them rely primarily on self-reported behavior. This is a limitation in that information about financial performance provided by the individual being assessed may reflect that person's lack of awareness of his or her impairment or deliberate efforts to conceal it. While some of these instruments show good psychometric properties in relation to other assessment methods, sufficient data on reliability and validity across populations are not yet available to warrant recommending their routine use.
- Although SSA provides field officers with a list of topic areas and questions to guide the in-person interviews with beneficiaries, many beneficiaries assessed for capability are not seen in person in a field office.
- Providing detailed guidance to all informants about the information on financial performance that SSA would find helpful in rendering a capability determination would likely improve the strength, quality, and consistency of the evidence it receives.

Financial Competence

- At times, no or very limited information about a beneficiary's financial performance will be available—for example, when the person has had no funds to manage or when no third-party informant with knowledge of the person's performance can be identified. When evidence of financial performance is unavailable, capability determinations may need to be based on evidence of financial competence. Evidence of beneficiaries' degree of financial competence also can help inform interpretations of the evidence regarding beneficiaries' financial performance.
- As with financial performance, detailed guidance and sample questions aimed at the assessment of financial competence would assist informants in providing relevant information about beneficiaries' financial knowledge and judgment, and would be likely to improve the strength, quality, and consistency of the evidence provided to SSA.
- As with instruments aimed at assessing financial performance, sufficient data on the reliability and validity across populations of

instruments for the assessment of financial competence are not yet available to warrant recommending their routine use.

Recommendation 1. The U.S. Social Security Administration (SSA) should provide detailed guidance to professional and lay informants regarding the information it would find most helpful for making capability determinations, including (1) information about specific aspects of beneficiaries' financial performance in meeting their basic needs and, when information about performance is unavailable, about their financial competence; and (2) information that would enable SSA to judge the validity of the evidence provided by the informant.

With respect to financial performance, SSA guidance to all medical and nonmedical informants could be based on the questions SSA currently provides to field officers (see Box 2-2 in Chapter 2). Additional questions, such as those included in the Financial Incapability Structured Clinical Assessment done Longitudinally (FISCAL), a financial performance assessment interview, may be helpful as well. Guidance pertaining to financial competence could include questions such as those developed by the Canada Pension Plan (see Box 5-1 in Chapter 5), along with requests that the basis for informants' answers be specified. Should sufficient data become available in the future on the reliability and validity of structured assessments of financial performance or competence, SSA guidance could be updated to indicate the value of such approaches. Asking informants to provide information based on a common set of questions in areas relevant to beneficiaries' financial performance and competence would help improve and standardize the information received by the field offices.

To enable SSA to judge the validity of information from informants, it is important that evidence provided for capability determinations specify how well and for how long the informant has known the individual and the nature of their relationship.[1] It is also important to specify the extent to which (1) the informant's judgment is based on observed behavior;[2] (2) the informant's judgment is based on the individual's self-report; (3) the informant's judgment is based on information from collateral informants, and the perceived quality of these informants; and (4) in the case of professionals,

---

[1] This would include, to the extent possible, the beneficiary's perspective on the relationship as well as the informant's.

[2] The U.S. Office of Personnel Management (OPM) asks informants to provide information about their "relationship to, and amount of contact with, the individual during the relevant time period" and "what actions or incidents were personally observed which would show whether the individual's condition interfered with the ability to handle personal affairs, and how often these were observed" (see Appendix C, OPM, Form RI 30-3, Information Necessary for Competency Determination).

the judgment is based on the individual's medical record and the assessments of other health care professionals (including other physicians, psychologists, social workers, and nurses). Such specification of the basis for the evidence provided will allow for greater understanding of the quality of the evidence as support for a judgment regarding financial capability.

It is important to note that personal and environmental factors may change or fluctuate, thereby affecting an individual's financial performance. For this reason, it is necessary not only to assess financial performance at a single point in time but also to assess it longitudinally to best estimate a person's financial capability. In addition, interpretations of evidence regarding beneficiaries' financial performance can be informed by evidence of beneficiaries' degree of financial competence.

SYSTEMATIC IDENTIFICATION OF ADULT SSA BENEFICIARIES AT RISK FOR FINANCIAL INCAPABILITY

Risk Criteria

The following conclusions and recommendations address systematic identification of individuals who are at risk for financial incapability.

- The primary goal of representative payment is to ensure that beneficiaries' basic needs—housing, food, and clothing—are being met. Research suggests beneficiaries with representative payees experience substantive benefits relative to their basic needs and improved substance abuse outcomes. For this reason, it is important that SSA identify potentially incapable beneficiaries to evaluate and make a determination regarding their capability.
- Multiple reviews by the SSA Office of the Inspector General (SSA-OIG) have suggested that SSA's current process for determining capability may be identifying too few beneficiaries who would benefit from a representative payee. Anecdotal evidence presented to the committee in open session suggests that SSA's capability determinations are more likely to miss beneficiaries who need a representative payee than to require a representative payee unnecessarily.
- Except for a limited number of conditions (e.g., coma lasting at least 30 days; verbal, performance, or full-scale intelligence quotient [IQ] of 59 or less), SSA currently has no standardized process for identifying individuals who may be in need of a capability evaluation.
- Reliance on diagnostic criteria alone to identify beneficiaries who need a representative payee is inadequate for a number of reasons,

including the likelihood of identifying too many people for capability evaluation in some diagnostic categories and missing people in other categories.

- Identification and development of easy-to-apply, efficient approaches, including screening criteria, that could be incorporated into the disability application process to identify people at high risk for incapability would be valuable in helping to ensure that potentially incapable beneficiaries receive further evaluation. Such approaches or criteria also could help identify recipients of old-age and retirement benefits who are at risk for financial incapability.

Recommendation 2. The U.S. Social Security Administration should create a data-driven process to support the development of approaches, including screening criteria, for identifying people at high risk for financial incapability.

SSA has the opportunity, whether through the development of formal screening criteria or other approaches (e.g., identifying risk markers to inform the judgment of field officers), to improve its ability to identify beneficiaries who may lack financial capability. The committee envisions the development of a model based on existing data, such as age, gender, impairment code, and education level, to identify predictors of incapability. The resulting model could be refined and its reliability and validity improved through pilot projects involving samples of beneficiaries who would undergo more detailed assessments of capability. Prior to large-scale implementation, the success of the resulting approach in identifying incapable beneficiaries who would otherwise not have been found could be tested.

Dual Beneficiaries

- A 2012 SSA-OIG report indicated that more than 6,000 individuals who were receiving benefits from both the Supplemental Security Income and Social Security Disability Insurance programs had been assigned a representative payee in one program but not the other.
- SSA beneficiaries also may receive benefits from another federal agency, such as the U.S. Department of Veterans Affairs (VA) or OPM, each of which has its own policies and procedures for determining whether beneficiaries are capable of managing their benefits.
- While acknowledging the potential technological, legal, and procedural challenges to data sharing, the committee concludes that sharing information about incapability determinations within SSA and among relevant federal agencies could increase the likelihood

of each agency's identifying potentially incapable beneficiaries. Agencies could use the information to trigger their own capability assessments of beneficiaries identified in this way.

Recommendation 3. The U.S. Social Security Administration (SSA) should ensure intra-agency communication regarding capability determinations within its different programs. In addition, SSA, the U.S. Department of Veterans Affairs, and other relevant federal agencies should assess the extent of inconsistency in the identification of beneficiaries who are incapable among persons receiving benefits from more than one agency. Based on the findings of this assessment, the relevant agencies should explore mechanisms to facilitate ongoing interagency communication regarding the capability of beneficiaries.

OPM, for example, uses computerized matching to identify beneficiaries who receive other federal benefits. Although such matching is used primarily to analyze whether benefits from other programs may affect OPM benefits, a process of this sort can also provide information that indicates whether other programs have identified the beneficiary as having impaired capability.

RESPONDING TO CHANGES IN CAPABILITY OVER TIME

The following conclusions and recommendation address the need for periodic reassessment of beneficiaries' financial capability over time.

- Many psychiatric and cognitive conditions are characterized by progression or fluctuation over time in the presence, severity, and nature of symptoms. Such changes suggest the value of a process for periodic reassessment of a beneficiary's capability.
- SSA's lack of a formal process for periodically reviewing a beneficiary's capability is a significant weakness. Some mechanism for periodic reassessment is needed to ensure that beneficiaries with fluctuating, deteriorating, or improving financial capability are classified accurately.

Recommendation 4. The U.S. Social Security Administration should develop systematic mechanisms for recognizing and responding to changes in beneficiaries' capability over time.

For disability beneficiaries, SSA procedures call for periodic continuing disability reviews (CDRs). Although CDRs provide an opportunity for capability (re)assessments, their purpose is to identify any changes (improvements) in the medical basis for beneficiaries' disability award. Thus, even if the CDRs were to occur on schedule, they would not fully serve the purpose of reassessment of financial capability.[3] SSA could apply the same principle used in the CDR process to develop an analogous process for recognizing and responding to changes in capability over time. Reassessments initially could be targeted toward (1) beneficiaries who had been determined to be incapable but who might improve over time as their conditions or environmental supports changed; and (2) beneficiaries who, although capable, were at risk for becoming incapable as their condition progressed or their environment changed. As screening criteria or other systematic methods for identifying people at high risk for financial incapability were developed, they might be used to broaden the target population for periodic reassessment.

In addition, beneficiaries, family members, representative payees, and professionals who were likely to come into contact with beneficiaries could be alerted systematically to notify SSA if they believed that beneficiaries' capability had changed so as to warrant redetermination. SSA might also implement a process to survey payees and/or beneficiaries periodically, similar to that of OPM, integrating screening questions that could trigger the need to further investigate the beneficiary's financial capability.

INNOVATION AND EVALUATION

Supervised Direct Payment

- The decision to appoint a representative payee affects the beneficiary's autonomy, and hence should occur only when clearly necessary to ensure that the beneficiary's basic needs will be met.
- When information available about a beneficiary's financial performance is insufficient to determine the need to appoint a representative payee, the use of a supervised direct payment option may be helpful. Under such a model, benefits are paid directly to the beneficiary, but an individual is designated to supervise the beneficiary's expenditures. Reassessment after a trial period during which the beneficiary's use of benefits is observed and assessed permits more accurate determination of the beneficiary's capability in indeterminate or borderline cases.

---

[3] For example, there are beneficiaries whose condition precludes their ability for substantial gainful activity but does not (yet) affect their financial competence or performance. When such a condition invariably will worsen, a CDR is required only every 5 to 7 years because the individual is not expected to regain the ability to work. As some of the conditions worsen, however, they may affect the individual's financial capability. Such cases are among those that are important for SSA to reevaluate.

- Supervised direct payment may have other advantages. By adopting a supported decision-making model, supervisors can provide guidance and instruction to beneficiaries on managing their benefits and help respond to the challenges posed by the fluctuations in some beneficiaries' financial competence and performance. Supported decision making encourages beneficiaries' expression of preferences, beliefs, and values; allows collaboration in decision making; and provides opportunities for beneficiaries to make independent decisions whenever possible. Appropriate use of this approach may provide a beneficiary with greater control over his or her life than would be the case for someone without such support.
- Supervised direct payment may enable some beneficiaries who might otherwise require the appointment of a representative payee to manage or direct the management of their benefits to meet their basic needs, thus maximizing their decisional autonomy.

Recommendation 5. The U.S. Social Security Administration should implement a demonstration project to evaluate the efficacy of a supervised direct payment option for qualified beneficiaries.

"Qualified beneficiaries" refers to two groups of individuals. The first is beneficiaries who may be incapable of managing or directing the management of their benefits but for whom there is insufficient information regarding financial performance to render a determination. The second is beneficiaries who are determined by SSA to be incapable, but who either display financial performance in some but not all areas of managing their benefits or successfully manage their benefits some but not all of the time. The VA's supervised direct payment option for individuals who are determined to be incompetent but able to manage benefits with supervision provides a model for such an approach. Instead of the VA's appointing a fiduciary for such individuals, they receive their benefits directly but under the supervision of a Veterans Service Center Manager. This approach could provide a model for a demonstration project by SSA.

Program Evaluation

- For the benefit programs examined by the committee, including SSA's, empirical data are lacking on the reliability and validity of capability/competency determinations, precluding assessment of the accuracy and efficiency of their determination processes.
- The committee has made a number of recommendations that could increase the accuracy of identification of beneficiaries in need of representative payees. Without baseline data and ongoing data

collection, however, the effectiveness of current policies or the impact of the recommended changes cannot be evaluated.

Recommendation 6. The U.S. Social Security Administration should develop and implement an ongoing measurement and evaluation process to quantify and track the accuracy of capability determinations and to inform and improve its policies and procedures for identifying beneficiaries who are incapable of managing or directing the management of their benefits.

The measurement and evaluation process envisioned in the present report would need to be designed and carried out by trained experts (whether in house or external) with detailed knowledge of SSA work flow and procedures. Such a process could comprise a variety of steps, including assessments of the interrater reliability of the capability determination process, in-depth assessments of selected beneficiaries to determine the accuracy of earlier determinations, and evaluations of the impact of the recommendations in this report (e.g., guidance on the evidence to be provided for capability determinations). A robust measurement and evaluation process would provide substantial and much-needed insight into what SSA is currently doing well and what it may, at reasonable cost, be able to do significantly better.

Appendix A

Public Session Agendas

MEETING 1: PUBLIC SESSION

Hosted by the Committee to Evaluate the Social Security Administration's Capability Determination Process for Adult Beneficiaries

February 3, 2014

Keck Center of the National Academies, Room 101
500 Fifth Street, NW
Washington, DC 20001

Agenda

10:30 a.m. **Welcome and Introductions**
Paul Appelbaum, M.D., Committee Chair

10:45 a.m. **Social Security Administration (SSA) Presentations Relevant to the Committee's Task**

Opening Remarks and Overview of the SSA Capability Determination Process
Shirleeta Stanton, Associate Commissioner, Office of Income Security Programs

	Description of the Capability Determination Process and the Field Office Role in the Process *Ann-Maria Beard,* Deputy Director, Office of Prisoner, Claimant, and Representative Payee Policy
	Description of the Disability Determination Services' Role in the Capability Determination Process *Dina Payne,* Policy Analyst, Office of Vocational, Evaluation, and Process Policy
11:30 a.m.	**Discussion of Statement of Task** Committee Members and SSA Staff
12:30 p.m.	**Break for Lunch**
1:30 p.m.	**Stakeholder Presentations and Discussion with Committee**
	National Alliance on Mental Illness *Andrew Sperling, J.D.,* Director of Federal Legislative Advocacy
	Judge David L. Bazelon Center for Mental Health Law *Ira A. Burnim, Esq.,* Legal Director
	Alzheimer's Association *Joan Quinn,* Interim Executive Director of the Connecticut (CT) Chapter and Interim Executive Director for the National Capital Area Chapter
3:25 p.m.	**Summary and Closing Remarks** *Paul Appelbaum, M.D.,* Committee Chair
3:30 p.m.	**Adjourn**

TELECONFERENCE WITH REPRESENTATIVES FROM THE NATIONAL ASSOCIATION OF DISABILITY EXAMINERS (NADE)

Hosted by the Committee to Evaluate the Social Security Administration's Capability Determination Process for Adult Beneficiaries

March 25, 2015

Keck Center of the National Academies, Room 400
500 Fifth Street, NW
Washington, DC 20001

Agenda

1:00 p.m. **Opening Remarks**
Paul Appelbaum, M.D., Committee Chair

Discussion with NADE representatives
Jeff Price, NADE President
Sharon Summers, NADE President-elect
Jennifer Nottingham, NADE Past President

2:00 p.m. **Adjourn**

MEETING 2: FINANCIAL CAPABILITY DETERMINATION PROCESSES

Hosted by the Committee to Evaluate the Social Security Administration's Capability Determination Process for Adult Beneficiaries

April 21, 2015

Keck Center of the National Academies, Room 208
500 Fifth Street, NW
Washington, DC 20001

Agenda

8:30 a.m. **Opening Remarks**
Paul Appelbaum, M.D., Committee Chair

8:40 a.m. **Assessing Financial Capacity: A Brief Overview**
Daniel C. Marson, J.D., Ph.D., Professor of Neurology; Director, Division of Neuropsychology; Director, Alzheimer's Disease Center, University of Alabama, Birmingham

9:55 a.m. **Break**

10:10 a.m. **Measuring Everyday Decision-Making Capacity**
Jason Karlawish, M.D., Professor of Medicine, Medical Ethics & Health Policy, University of Pennsylvania

11:05 a.m. **Data-Driven Approaches to Assessing Which SSI/SSDI Recipients Are Capable of Managing Their Benefits**
Marc I. Rosen, Ph.D., Associate Professor of Psychiatry, Yale, New Haven, Connecticut; Staff Psychiatrist, Veterans Affairs Connecticut

12:00 p.m. **Break for Lunch**

1:00 p.m. **Presentation and Discussion of the U.S. Department of Veterans Affairs Process for Capability Determination**
Brad Flohr, Senior Advisor for Compensation Service, U.S. Department of Veterans Affairs

Cynthia Lewis, Chief, Pension and Fiduciary Service, U.S. Department of Veterans Affairs

2:55 p.m. **Closing Remarks**
Paul Appelbaum, M.D., Committee Chair

3:00 p.m. **Adjourn**

MEETING 3: FINANCIAL CAPABILITY DETERMINATION PROCESSES

Hosted by the Committee to Evaluate the Social Security Administration's Capability Determination Process for Adult Beneficiaries

June 24, 2015

Keck Center of the National Academies, Room 201
500 Fifth Street, NW
Washington, DC 20001

Agenda

9:00 a.m.	**Opening Remarks** *Paul Appelbaum, M.D.*, Committee Chair
9:15 a.m.	**The Representative Payee System, Process, and Impacts on the Beneficiary** Moderator—*Julie Birkenmaier, Ph.D., M.S.W., LCSW*, Committee Member *Eric Elbogen, Ph.D.*, Associate Professor, Forensic Psychiatry Program and Clinic, University of North Carolina at Chapel Hill *Wendy Guyton, LICSW*, Social Services Supervisor, Bread for the City, Washington, DC *David Freeman, Psy.D.*, Associate Director for Assertive Community Treatment (ACT), Community Connections, Washington, DC
11:15 a.m.	**Break**
11:30 a.m.	**Representative Payee Process** *Quinta Spear, Ph.D.*, Deputy Assistant Director, DC, Retirement Operations, U.S. Office of Personnel Management
12:15 p.m.	**Break for Lunch**

1:15 p.m. **Abilities Required to Manage or Direct the Management of Benefits: Conceptual and Applied**
Moderator—*Laura B. Dunn, M.D.*, Committee Member

Stacey Wood, Ph.D., Clinical Psychologist and Associate Professor of Psychology, Scripps College, Claremont, California

Peter Lichtenberg, Ph.D., Director, Institute of Gerontology; Director, Merrill Palmer Skillman Institute; Professor of Psychology, Wayne State University, Detroit, Michigan

2:45 p.m. **Break**

3:00 p.m. **Effects of Everyday Surroundings and Pressures on Capability**
Eldar Shafir, Ph.D., William Stewart Tod Professor of Psychology and Public Affairs, Princeton University, New Jersey

4:00 p.m. **Closing Remarks**
Paul Appelbaum, M.D., Committee Chair

TELECONFERENCE WITH REPRESENTATIVES FROM SERVICE CANADA

Hosted by the Committee to Evaluate the Social Security Administration's Capability Determination Process for Adult Beneficiaries

October 9, 2015

National Academy of Sciences Building, Board Room
2101 Constitution Avenue, NW
Washington, DC 20418

Agenda

10:30 a.m. **Opening Remarks**
Paul Appelbaum, M.D., Committee Chair

Discussion with Representatives from Service Canada
Michael A. Kidd, Executive Director, Canada Pension Plan and Old Age Security Business Operations

11:00 a.m. **Adjourn**

Appendix B

Glossary

Ability: The power or skill to do something; the quality or state of being able, especially physical, mental, or legal power to perform; competence in doing; natural aptitude or acquired proficiency (Merriam-Webster, 2015).

Capability (U.S. Social Security Administration [SSA]): "Capability refers to a beneficiary's ability to manage or direct the management of his [or] her Social Security funds. . . . A beneficiary who exercises direct involvement, control and choice in identifying, accessing and managing services to meet his/her personal and other needs is capable and must be paid directly" (SSA, 2015b).

Financial capability: The management or direction of the management of one's funds in a way that routinely meets one's best interests.

Financial competence: The financial knowledge and skills one possesses. It includes both financial knowledge and financial judgment (defined below).

Financial incapability: Inability to manage or direct the management of one's funds in a way that meets one's basic needs and goals. May be manifest by a failure to demonstrate financial performance, as defined above, routinely.

Financial judgment: Possession of the abilities needed to make financial decisions and choices that serve the individual's best interests.

Financial knowledge: Possession of the declarative and procedural knowledge required to manage one's finances.

Financial literacy: "The knowledge and skills needed to make sound financial decisions" (Collins, 2013, p. 1).

Financial performance: The degree of success in handling financial demands in the context of the stresses, supports, contextual cues, and resources in the individual's actual environment. A high degree of financial performance requires not only sufficient levels of financial competence, but also possession of the skills needed to implement financial decisions in everyday life and the opportunity to exercise those skills.

Incompetency (legal): A determination by the courts that an individual is unable to manage his or her affairs as a result of mental deficiency or, sometimes, physical disability. The U.S. Social Security Administration uses the term "legally incompetent" to refer to one subset of beneficiaries who will automatically receive a representative payee.

Lay evidence (SSA): "Lay evidence is anything other than legal or medical evidence, which gives insight into a beneficiary's ability to manage or direct the management of his/her funds" (SSA, 2015d). Sources of lay evidence may include U.S. Social Security Administration employees; nonprofessionals (e.g., relatives, friends, neighbors); and health care and other professionals (e.g., social workers, occupational therapists, rehabilitation specialists, adult protective services workers).

Legal evidence (SSA): "Legal evidence is one type of evidence that establishes an individual's ability to handle his/her financial affairs. There must be a court order in place for a finding that an individual is incompetent. . . . The court order must specifically address the beneficiary's competency or must contain a statement regarding the individual's ability to handle his/her financial affairs" (SSA, 2015a).

Medical evidence (SSA): "Medical evidence of capability is evidence of a medical nature that sheds light on a beneficiary's ability to manage or direct the management of funds. The term, 'of a medical nature,' means from a physician, psychologist or other qualified medical practitioner who is in a position to provide a meaningful assessment of the beneficiary's ability to manage funds. . . . Acceptable medical evidence is an opinion offered by a medical professional (e.g., physician, psychologist), based on an examination of the beneficiary" (SSA, 2015c).

Representative payee (SSA): "A person designated by the Social Security Administration to receive monthly benefit checks on behalf of a beneficiary who is unable to manage his or her own funds" (SSA, 2014).

REFERENCES

Collins, J. M. 2013. Analyzing the financial capability of people in Wisconsin. *Issue briefs: Family financial education 2013-04*. http://fyi.uwex.edu/financialseries/files/2013/04/April_2013_Fin_Cap1.pdf (accessed September 11, 2015).

Merriam-Webster. 2015. Ability. *Merriam-Webster Dictionary* [online]. http://www.merriam-webster.com/dictionary/ability (accessed August 11, 2015).

SSA (U.S. Social Security Administration). 2014. *Annual statistical report on the Social Security Disability Insurance Program, 2013*. SSA Publication No. 13-11826. Washington, DC: SSA. http://www.ssa.gov/policy/docs/statcomps/di_asr/2013/di_asr13.pdf (accessed August 4, 2015).

SSA. 2015a. *GN 00502.005 Direct payment prohibitions*. https://secure.ssa.gov/poms.nsf/lnx/0200502005 (accessed August 4, 2015).

SSA. 2015b. *GN 00502.010 Capability determination—overview*. https://secure.ssa.gov/poms.nsf/lnx/0200502010 (accessed August 4, 2015).

SSA. 2015c. *GN 00502.025 Medical evidence of capability*. https://secure.ssa.gov/poms.nsf/lnx/0200502025 (accessed August 4, 2015).

SSA. 2015d. *GN 00502.030 Lay evidence of capability*. https://secure.ssa.gov/poms.nsf/lnx/0200502030 (accessed August 4, 2015).

Appendix C

Selected Forms

SOCIAL SECURITY ADMINISTRATION TOE 250 Form Approved OMB No. 0960-0024

PHYSICIAN'S/MEDICAL OFFICER'S STATEMENT OF PATIENT'S CAPABILITY TO MANAGE BENEFITS

Paperwork Reduction Act Statement - This information collection meets the requirements of 44 U.S.C. § 3507, as amended by Section 2 of the Paperwork Reduction Act of 1995. You do not need to answer these questions unless we display a valid Office of Management and Budget control number. We estimate that it will take about 10 minutes to read the instructions, gather the facts, and answer the questions. **SEND OR BRING THE COMPLETED FORM TO YOUR LOCAL SOCIAL SECURITY OFFICE. You can find your local Social Security office through SSA's website at** www.socialsecurity.gov. **Offices are also listed under U.S. Government agencies in your telephone directory or you may call Social Security at 1-800-772-1213 (TTY 1-800-325-0778).** ***Send only comments relating to our time estimate above to:*** *SSA, 6401 Security Blvd, Baltimore, MD 21235-6401.*

In replying, use this address:
SOCIAL SECURITY ADMINISTRATION

TELEPHONE NUMBER (Including Area Code)
(   )   -

DATE

SSA CONTACT

IDENTIFYING INFORMATION (SSA Only)
If different from patient

NAME OF WAGE EARNER OR SELF-EMPLOYED PERSON

SOCIAL SECURITY NUMBER
-    -

Privacy Act Statement

Sections 205(a) and 205(j), of the Social Security Act, as amended, authorize us to collect this information. The information is needed to make a determination regarding whether or not the named individual should be paid benefits directly or whether benefits should be paid to a representative payee. The information you furnish on this form is voluntary. However, failure to provide all or part of the information could prevent an accurate and timely decision on the proper payee for benefit receipt purposes.

We rarely use the information you supply for any purpose other than for making a determination on a claim. However, we may use it for the administration and integrity of Social Security programs. We may also disclose information to another person or to another agency in accordance with approved routine uses, which include but are not limited to: (1) to enable a third party or an agency to assist Social Security in establishing rights to Social Security benefits and/or coverage; (2) to comply with Federal laws requiring the release of information from Social Security records (e.g., to the Government Accountability Office and Department of Veteran Affairs); (3) to make determinations for eligibility in similar health and income maintenance programs at the Federal, state, and local level; and (4) to facilitate statistical research, audit or investigative activities necessary to assure the integrity of Social Security programs.

We may also use the information you provide in computer matching programs. Matching programs compare our records with records kept by other Federal, state or local government agencies. Information from these matching programs can be used to establish or verify a person's eligibility for Federally funded and administered benefit programs and for repayment of payments or delinquent debts under these programs.

A complete list of routine uses for this information is available in Systems of Record Notices 60-0089 and 60-0222. The notices, additional information regarding this form, and information regarding our programs and systems, are available on-line at www.socialsecurity.gov or at your local Social Security office.

PATIENT'S NAME		PATIENT'S ADDRESS (Number and Street, City, State, and ZIP Code)
PATIENT'S SOCIAL SECURITY NUMBER - -	PATIENT'S DATE OF BIRTH	

YOUR HELP IS NEEDED

The patient shown above has filed for or is receiving Social Security or Supplemental Security Income payments. We need you to complete the back of this form and return it to us in the enclosed envelope to help us decide if we should pay this person directly or if he or she needs a representative payee to handle the funds. Please Note: This determination affects how benefits are paid and has no bearing on disability determinations; SSA will NOT pay for this information. Thank you for your help.

WHO IS A REPRESENTATIVE PAYEE

A representative payee is someone who manages the patient's money to make sure the patient's needs are met. The payee has a strong and continuing interest in the patient's well-being and is usually a family member or close friend.

WHO NEEDS A REPRESENTATIVE PAYEE

Some individuals age 18 and older who have mental or physical impairments are not capable of handling their funds or directing others how to handle them to meet their basic needs, so we select a representative payee to receive their payments. Examples of impairments which may cause incapability are senility, severe brain damage or chronic schizophrenia. However, even though a person may need some assistance with such things as bill paying, etc., does not necessarily mean he/she cannot make decisions concerning basic needs and is incapable of managing his/her own money.

PLEASE COMPLETE THE INFORMATION ON THE REVERSE OF THIS FORM

Form **SSA-787** (05-2010) ef (05-2010) Destroy Prior Editions

PHYSICIAN'S/MEDICAL OFFICER'S STATEMENT OF PATIENT'S CAPABILITY TO MANAGE BENEFITS

Paperwork Reduction Act Statement - This information collection meets the requirements of 44 U.S.C. § 3507, as amended by Section 2 of the Paperwork Reduction Act of 1995. You do not need to answer these questions unless we display a valid Office of Management and Budget control number. We estimate that it will take about 10 minutes to read the instructions, gather the facts, and answer the questions. **SEND OR BRING THE COMPLETED FORM TO YOUR LOCAL SOCIAL SECURITY OFFICE. You can find your local Social Security office through SSA's website at** www.socialsecurity.gov. **Offices are also listed under U.S. Government agencies in your telephone directory or you may call Social Security at 1-800-772-1213 (TTY 1-800-325-0778).** ***Send only comments relating to our time estimate above to:*** *SSA, 6401 Security Blvd, Baltimore, MD 21235-6401.*

In replying, use this address:
SOCIAL SECURITY ADMINISTRATION

TELEPHONE NUMBER (Including Area Code)
(   )   -

DATE

SSA CONTACT

Privacy Act Statement

Sections 205(a) and 205(j), of the Social Security Act, as amended, authorize us to collect this information. The information is needed to make a determination regarding whether or not the named individual should be paid benefits directly or whether benefits should be paid to a representative payee. The information you furnish on this form is voluntary. However, failure to provide all or part of the information could prevent an accurate and timely decision on the proper payee for benefit receipt purposes.

We rarely use the information you supply for any purpose other than for making a determination on a claim. However, we may use it for the administration and integrity of Social Security programs. We may also disclose information to another person or to another agency in accordance with approved routine uses, which include but are not limited to: (1) to enable a third party or an agency to assist Social Security in establishing rights to Social Security benefits and/or coverage; (2) to comply with Federal laws requiring the release of information from Social Security records (e.g., to the Government Accountability Office and Department of Veteran Affairs); (3) to make determinations for eligibility in similar health and income maintenance programs at the Federal, state, and local level; and (4) to facilitate statistical research, audit or investigative activities necessary to assure the integrity of Social Security programs.

We may also use the information you provide in computer matching programs. Matching programs compare our records with records kept by other Federal, state or local government agencies. Information from these matching programs can be used to establish or verify a person's eligibility for Federally funded and administered benefit programs and for repayment of payments or delinquent debts under these programs.

A complete list of routine uses for this information is available in Systems of Record Notices 60-0089 and 60-0222. The notices, additional information regarding this form, and information regarding our programs and systems, are available on-line at www.socialsecurity.gov or at your local Social Security office.

IDENTIFYING INFORMATION (SSA Only)
If different from patient

NAME OF WAGE EARNER OR SELF-EMPLOYED PERSON

SOCIAL SECURITY NUMBER
  - -

PATIENT'S NAME		PATIENT'S ADDRESS (Number and Street, City, State, and ZIP Code)
PATIENT'S SOCIAL SECURITY NUMBER - -	PATIENT'S DATE OF BIRTH	

YOUR HELP IS NEEDED

The patient shown above has filed for or is receiving Social Security or Supplemental Security Income payments. We need you to complete the back of this form and return it to us in the enclosed envelope to help us decide if we should pay this person directly or if he or she needs a representative payee to handle the funds. Please Note: This determination affects how benefits are paid and has no bearing on disability determinations; SSA will NOT pay for this information. Thank you for your help.

WHO IS A REPRESENTATIVE PAYEE

A representative payee is someone who manages the patient's money to make sure the patient's needs are met. The payee has a strong and continuing interest in the patient's well-being and is usually a family member or close friend.

WHO NEEDS A REPRESENTATIVE PAYEE

Some individuals age 18 and older who have mental or physical impairments are not capable of handling their funds or directing others how to handle them to meet their basic needs, so we select a representative payee to receive their payments. Examples of impairments which may cause incapability are senility, severe brain damage or chronic schizophrenia. However, even though a person may need some assistance with such things as bill paying, etc., does not necessarily mean he/she cannot make decisions concerning basic needs and is incapable of managing his/her own money.

PLEASE COMPLETE THE INFORMATION ON THE REVERSE OF THIS FORM

Form **SSA-787** (05-2010) ef (05-2010) Destroy Prior Editions

SOCIAL SECURITY ADMINISTRATION TOE 250 Form Approved OMB No. 0960-0014

REQUEST TO BE SELECTED AS PAYEE

FOR SSA USE ONLY							
Name or Bene. Sym.	Program	Date of Birth	Type	Gdn.	Cus.	Inst.	Nam.

FOR SSA USE ONLY

DISTRICT OFFICE CODE

STATE AND COUNTY CODE

PRINT IN INK:

The name of the NUMBER HOLDER	SOCIAL SECURITY NUMBER
The name of the PERSON(S) (if different from above) for whom you are filing (the "claimant(s)")	SOCIAL SECURITY NUMBER(S)

Answer item 1 ONLY if you are the claimant and want your benefits paid directly to you.

1. I request that I be paid directly.
CHECK HERE ☐ and answer only items 3, 5, 6, and 8 before signing the form on page 4.

I REQUEST THAT THE SOCIAL SECURITY, SUPPLEMENTAL SECURITY INCOME, OR SPECIAL VETERANS BENEFITS FOR THE CLAIMANT(S) NAMED ABOVE BE PAID TO ME AS REPRESENTATIVE PAYEE.

2. Explain why you think the claimant is not able to handle his/her own benefits. (In your answer, describe how he/she manages any money he/she receives now.)

☐ Claimant is a minor child

3. Explain why you would be the best representative payee. (Use Remarks if you need more space.)

4. If you are appointed payee, how will you know about the claimant's needs?

☐ Live with me or in the institution I represent

☐ Daily visits

☐ Visits at least once a week.

☐ By other means. Explain:

5. Does the claimant have a court-appointed legal guardian/conservator? ☐ YES ☐ NO

IF YES, enter the legal guardian/conservator's:

NAME ______________________

ADDRESS ______________________

PHONE NUMBER ______________________

TITLE ______________________

DATE OF APPOINTMENT ______________________

Explain the circumstances of the appointment. (Use remarks if you need more space.)

Form **SSA-11-BK** (01-2014) EF (01-2014) Page 1
Use (08-2009) EF (08-2009) edition until exhausted

6. (a) Where does the claimant live?

- [ ] Alone
- [ ] In my home (Go to (b).)
- [ ] With a relative (Go to (b).)
- [ ] With someone else (Go to (b).)
- [ ] In a board and care facility (Go to (b).)
- [ ] In a public institution (Go to (c).)
- [ ] In a private institution (Go to (c).)
- [ ] In a nursing home (Go to (c).)
- [ ] In the institution I represent (Go to (c).)

(b) Enter the names and relationships of any other people who live with the claimant.

NAME	RELATIONSHIP

(c) Enter the claimant's residence and mailing addresses (if different from yours).

Residence: Mailing: Telephone Number:

(d) Do you expect the claimant's living arrangements to change in the next year?

☐ YES ☐ NO If YES, explain what changes are expected and when they will occur. (Use Remarks if you need more space.)

7. If you are applying on behalf of minor child(ren) and you are not the parent,

Does the child(ren) have a living natural or adoptive parent? ☐ YES ☐ NO

If YES, enter: (a) Name of parent ____________

(b) Address of parent ____________

(c) Telephone number ____________

(d) Does the parent show interest in the child? ☐ YES ☐ NO

Please explain. ____________

8. List the names and relationship of any (other) relatives or close friends who have provided support and/or show active interest with the claimant. Describe the type and amount of support and/or how interest is displayed.

NAME	ADDRESS/PHONE NO.	RELATIONSHIP	DESCRIBE

9. Check the block that describes your relationship to the claimant.

(a) ☐ Official of bank, agency or institution with responsibility for the person. Enter below which you represent:

- [ ] Bank
- [ ] Social Agency
- [ ] Public Official
- [ ] Institution:
  - [ ] Federal
  - [ ] State/Local
  - [ ] Private non-profit
  - [ ] Private proprietary institution. Is the institution licensed under State law? ☐ YES ☐ NO

IF (a) ABOVE CHECKED, COMPLETE ONLY QUESTIONS 10 AND 11 AND SIGN THE FORM ON PAGE 4.

(b) ☐ Parent

(c) ☐ Spouse

(d) ☐ Other Relative - Specify

(e) ☐ Legal Representative

(f) ☐ Board and Care Home Operator

(g) ☐ Other Individual - Specify

IF (b), (c), (d), or (e) ABOVE CHECKED, GO ON TO QUESTION 12

10. Does the claimant owe you/your organization any money now or will he/she owe you money in the future?
☐ YES ☐ NO

If YES, enter the amount he/she owes you/your organization, the date(s) was/will be incurred and describe why the debt was/will be incurred.

INFORMATION ABOUT INSTITUTIONS, AGENCIES AND BANKS APPLYING TO BE REPRESENTATIVE PAYEE

11. (a) Enter the name of the institution ______

(b) Enter the EIN of the institution ______

INFORMATION ABOUT INDIVIDUALS APPLYING TO BE REPRESENTATIVE PAYEE

12. Enter: YOUR NAME ______

DATE OF BIRTH ______

SOCIAL SECURITY NUMBER ______

ANY OTHER NAME YOU HAVE USED ______

OTHER SSN'S YOU HAVE USED ______

13. How long have you known the claimant? ______

14. If the claimant lives with you, who takes care of the claimant when work or other activity takes you away from home?

What is his/her relationship to the claimant?

15. (a) Main source of your income

- ☐ Employed (answer (b) below)
- ☐ Self-employed (Type of Business ______)
- ☐ Social Security benefits (Claim Number ______)
- ☐ Pension (describe ______)
- ☐ Supplemental Security Income payments (Claim Number ______)
- ☐ AFDC (County & State ______)
- ☐ Other Welfare (describe ______)
- ☐ Other (describe ______)

(b) Enter your employer's name and address:

How long have you been employed by this employer? ______
(If less than 1 year, enter name and address of previous employer in Remarks.)

16. (a) Have you ever been convicted of a felony? ☐ YES ☐ NO

If YES: What was the crime? ______

On what date were you convicted? ______

What was your sentence? ______

If imprisoned, when were you released? ______

If probation was ordered, when did/will your probation end? ______

(b) Have you ever been convicted of any offense under federal or state law which resulted in imprisonment for more than one year? ☐ YES ☐ NO

If YES: What was the crime? ______

On what date were you convicted? ______

What was your sentence? ______

If imprisoned, when were you released? ______

If probation was ordered, when did/will your probation end? ______

17.	Do you have any unsatisfied FELONY warrants (or in jurisdictions that do not define crimes as felonies, a crime punishable by death or imprisonment exceeding 1 year) for your arrest? ☐ YES ☐ NO If YES: Date of Warrant ________ State where warrant was issued ________
18.	How long have you lived at your current address? (Give Date MM/YY)

REMARKS: *(This space may be used for explaining any answers to the questions. If you need more space, attach a separate sheet.)*

PLEASE READ THE FOLLOWING INFORMATION CAREFULLY BEFORE SIGNING THIS FORM

I/my organization:
- Must use all payments made to me/my organization as the representative payee for the claimant's current needs or (if not currently needed) save them for his/her future needs.
- May be held liable for repayment if I/my organization misuse the payments or if I/my organization am/is at fault for any overpayment of benefits.
- May be punished under Federal law by fine, imprisonment or both if I/my organization am/is found guilty of misuse of Social Security or SSI benefits.

I/my organization will:
- Use the payments for the claimant's current needs and save any currently unneeded benefits for future use.
- File an accounting report on how the payments were used, and make all supporting records available for review if requested by the Social Security Administration.
- Reimburse the amount of any loss suffered by any claimant due to misuse of Social Security or SSI funds by me/my organization.
- Notify the Social Security Administration when the claimant dies, leaves my/my organization's custody or otherwise changes his/her living arrangements or he/she is no longer my/my organization's responsibility.
- Comply with the conditions for reporting certain events (listed on the attached sheets(s) which I/my organization will keep for my/my organization's records) and for returning checks the claimant is not due.
- File an annual report of earnings if required.
- Notify the Social Security Administration as soon as I/my organization can no longer act as representative payee or the claimant no longer needs a payee.

I declare under penalty of perjury that I have examined all the information on this form, and on any accompanying statements or forms, and it is true and correct to the best of my knowledge.

SIGNATURE OF APPLICANT	DATE *(Month, day, year)*
Signature *(First name, middle initial, last name) (Write in ink)*	Telephone number(s) at which you may be contacted during the day

Print Your Name & Title *(if a representative or employee of an institution/organization)*

Mailing Address *(Number and street, Apt. No., P.O. Box, or Rural Route)*

City and State	Zip Code	Name of County

Residence Address *(Number and street, Apt. No., P.O. Box, or Rural Route)*

City and State	Zip Code	Name of County

Witnesses are only required if this application has been signed by mark (X) above. If signed by mark (X), two witnesses to the signing who know the applicant making the request must sign below, giving their full addresses.

1. SIGNATURE OF WITNESS	2. SIGNATURE OF WITNESS
ADDRESS *(Number and street, City, State and ZIP Code)*	ADDRESS *(Number and street, City, State and ZIP Code)*

SOCIAL SECURITY
Information for Representative Payees Who Recieve Social Security Benefits

YOU MUST NOTIFY THE SOCIAL SECURITY ADMINISTRATION PROMPTLY IF ANY OF THE FOLLOWING EVENTS OCCUR AND PROMPTLY RETURN ANY PAYMENT TO WHICH THE CLAIMANT IS NOT ENTITLED:

- the claimant DIES (Social Security entitlement ends the month before the month the claimant dies);
- the claimant MARRIES, if the claimant is entitled to child's, widow's, mother's, father's, widower's or parent's benefits, or to wife's or husband's benefits as divorced wife/husband, or to special age 72 payments;
- the claimant's marriage ends in DIVORCE or ANNULMENT, if the claimant is entitled to wife's, husband's or special age 72 payments;
- the claimant's SCHOOL ATTENDANCE CHANGES if the claimant is age 18 or over and entitled to child's benefits as a full time student
- the claimant is entitled as a stepchild and the parents DIVORCE (benefits terminate the month after the month the divorce becomes final);
- the claimant is under FULL RETIREMENT AGE (FRA) and WORKS for more than the annual limit (as determined each year) or more than the allowable time (for work outside the United States);
- the claimant receives a GOVERNMENT PENSION or ANNUITY or the amount of the annuity changes, if the claimant is entitled to husband's, widower's, or divorced spouse's benefit's;
- the claimant leaves your custody or care or otherwise CHANGES ADDRESS;
- the claimant NO LONGER HAS A CHILD IN CARE, if he/she is entitled to benefits because of caring for a child under age 16 or who is disabled;
- the claimant is confined to jail, prison, penal institution or correctional facility;
- the claimant is confined to a public institution by court order in connection WITH A CRIME.
- the claimant has an UNSATISFIED FELONY WARRANT (or in jurisdictions that do not define crimes as felonies, a crime punishable by death or imprisonment exceeding 1 year) issue for his/her arrest;
- the claimant is violating a condition of probation or parole under State or Federal law.

IF THE CLAIMANT IS RECEIVING DISABILITY BENEFITS, YOU MUST ALSO REPORT IF:

- the claimant's MEDICAL CONDITION IMPROVES;
- the claimant STARTS WORKING;
- the claimant applies for or receives WORKER'S COMPENSATION BENEFITS, Black Lung Benefits from the Department of Labor, or a public disability benefit;
- the claimant is DISCHARGED FROM THE HOSPITAL (if now hospitalized).

IF THE CLAIMAINT IS RECEIVING SPECIAL AGE 72 PAYMENTS, YOU MUST ALSO REPORT IF:

- the claimant or spouse becomes ELIGIBLE FOR PERIODIC GOVERNMENTAL PAYMENTS, whether from the U.S. Federal government or from any State or local government;
- the claimant or spouse receives SUPPLEMENTAL SECURITY INCOME or PUBLIC ASSISTANCE CASH BENEFITS;
- the claimant or spouse MOVES outside the United States (the 50 States, the District of Columbia and the Northern Marian Islands).

In addition to these events about the claimant, you must also notify us if:

- YOU change your address;
- YOU are convicted of a felony or any offense under State or Federal law which results in imprisonment for more than 1 year;
- YOU have a UNSATISFIED FELONY WARRANT (or in jurisdictions that do not define crimes as felonies, a crime punishable by death or imprisonment exceeding 1 year) issued for your arrest.

BENEFITS MAY STOP IF ANY OF THE ABOVE EVENTS OCCUR. You should read the informational booklet we will send you to see how these events affect benefits. You may make your reports by telephone, mail, or in person.

REMEMBER:

- **payments must be used for the claimant's current needs or saved if not currently needed;**
- **you may be held liable for repayment of any payments not used for the claimant's needs or of any over payment that occured due to your fault;**
- **you must account for benefits when so asked by the Social Security Administration. You will keep records of how benefits were spent so you can provide us with correct accounting;**
- **to tell us as soon as you know you will no longer be able to act as representative payee or the claimant no longer needs a payee.**

Keep in mind that benefits may be deposited directly into an account set up for the claimant with you as payee. As soon as you set up such an account, contact us for more information about receiving the claimant's payments using direct deposit.

Form **SSA-11-BK** (01-2014) EF (01-2014) Page 5

A REMINDER TO PAYEE APPLICANTS

TELEPHONE NUMBER(S) TO CALL IF YOU HAVE A QUESTION OR SOMETHING TO REPORT	BEFORE YOU RECEIVE A DECISION NOTICE	SSA OFFICE	DATE REQUEST RECEIVED
	AFTER YOU RECEIVE A DECISION NOTICE		

RECEIPT FOR YOUR REQUEST

Your request for Social Security benefits on behalf of the individual(s) named below has been received and will be processed as quickly as possible.

You should hear from us within______ days after you have given us all the information we requested. Some claims may take longer if additional information is needed.

In the meantime, if you change your address, or if there is some other change that may affect the benefits payable, you - or someone for you - should report the change. The changes to be reported are listed on the reverse.

Always give us the claim number of the beneficiary when writing or telephoning about the claim.

If you have any questions about this application, we will be glad to help you.

BENEFICIARY	SOCIAL SECURITY CLAIM NUMBER

Privacy Act Statement - Collection and Use of Personal Information

Sections 205(a) and 205(j) of the Social Security Act, as amended, authorize us to collect this information. We will use the information you provide to determine if you are qualified to serve as a representative payee. Furnishing us this information is voluntary. However, failing to provide all or part of the information could prevent us from making a determination to select you as a representative payee.

We rarely use the information you supply for any purpose other than for determining continuing eligibility. However, we may use it for the administration and integrity of our programs. We may also disclose information to another person or to another agency in accordance with approved routine uses, which include but are not limited to the following: 1. To enable a third party or an agency to assist us in establishing rights to our benefits and coverage; 2. To comply with Federal laws requiring the release of information from our records (e.g., to the Government Accountability Office and Department of Veterans Affairs); 3. To make determinations for eligibility in similar health and income maintenance programs at the Federal, State, and local level; and, 4. To facilitate statistical research, audit, or investigative activities necessary to assure the integrity and improvement of our programs. (e.g., to the Bureau of Census and to private entities under contract with us).

We may also use the information you provide in computer matching programs. Matching programs compare our records with records kept by other Federal, State, or local government agencies. We use the information from these matching programs to establish or verify a person's eligibility for federally funded or administered benefit programs and for repayment of incorrect payments or delinquent debts under these programs.

A complete list of routine uses for this information is available in our Privacy Act Systems of Records Notice entitled, Master Representative Payee File, 60-0222. Additional information regarding these and other systems of records notices are available on-line at www.socialsecurity.gov or at your local Social Security office.

Paperwork Reduction Act Statement - This information collection meets the requirements of 44 U.S.C. § 3507, as amended by section 2 of the Paperwork Reduction Act of 1995. You do not need to answer these questions unless we display a valid Office of Management and Budget (OMB) control number. We estimate that it will take about 11 minutes to read the instructions, gather the facts, and answer the questions. ***Send only comments relating to our time estimate above to***: *SSA, 6401 Security Blvd, Baltimore, MD 21235-0001.*

SUPPLEMENTAL SECURITY INCOME
Information for Representative Payees Who Receive Social Security Benefits

YOU MUST NOTIFY THE SOCIAL SECURITY ADMINISTRATION PROMPTLY IF ANY OF THE FOLLOWING EVENTS OCCUR AND PROMPTLY RETURN ANY PAYMENT TO WHICH THE CLAIMANT IS NOT ENTITLED:

- the claimant or any member of the claimant's household DIES (SSI eligibility ends with the month in which the claimant dies);
- the claimant's HOUSEHOLD CHANGES (someone moves in/out of the place where the claimant lives);
- the claimant LEAVES THE U.S. (the 50 states, the District of Columbia, and the Northern Mariana Islands) for 30 consecutive days or more;
- the claimant MOVES or otherwise changes the place where he/she actually lives (including adoption, and whereabouts unknown);
- the claimant is ADMITTED TO A HOSPITAL, skilled nursing facility, nursing home, intermediate care facility, or other institution;
- the INCOME of the claimant or anyone in the claimant's household CHANGES (this includes income paid by an organization or employer, as well as monetary benefits from other sources);
- the RESOURCES of the claimant or anyone in the claimant's household CHANGES (this includes when conserved funds reach over $2,000);
- the claimant or anyone in the claimant's household MARRIES;
- the marriage of the claimant or anyone in the claimant's household ends in DIVORCE or ANNULMENT;
- the claimant SEPARATES from his/her spouse;
- the claimant is confined to jail, prison, penal institution or correctional facility;
- the claimant is confined to a public institution by court order in connection WITH A CRIME;
- the claimant has an UNSATISFIED FELONY WARRANT (or in jurisdictions that do not define crimes as felonies, a crime punishable by death or imprisonment exceeding 1 year) issued for his/her arrest;
- the claimant is violating a condition of probation or parole under State or Federal law.

IF THE CLAIMANT IS RECEIVING PAYMENTS DUE TO DISABILITY OR BLINDNESS, YOU MUST ALSO REPORT IF:

- the claimant's MEDICAL CONDITION IMPROVES;
- the claimant GOES TO WORK;
- the claimant's VISION IMPROVES, if the claimant is entitled due to blindness;

In addition to these events about the claimant, you must also notify us if:

- YOU change your address;
- YOU are convicted of a felony or any offense under State or Federal law which results in imprisonment for more than 1 year;
- YOU have an UNSATISFIED FELONY WARRANT (or in jurisdictions that do not define crimes as felonies, a crime punishable by death or imprisonment exceeding 1 year) issued for your arrest.

PAYMENT MAY STOP IF ANY OF THE ABOVE EVENTS OCCUR. You should read the informational booklet we will send you to see how these events affect benefits. You may make your reports by telephone, mail or in person.

REMEMBER :

- payments must be used for the claimant's current needs or saved if not currently needed. (Savings are considered resources and may affect the claimant's eligibility to payment.);
- you may be held liable for repayment of any payments not used for the claimant's needs or of any overpayment that occurred due to your fault;
- you must account for benefits when so asked by the Social Security Administration. You will keep records of how benefits were spent so you can provide us with a correct accounting;
- to let us know as soon as you know you are unable to continue as representative payee or the claimant no longer needs a payee
- you will be asked to help in periodically redetermining the claimant's continued eligibility or payment. You will need to keep evidence to help us with the redetermination (e.g., evidence of income and living arrangements).
- you may be required to obtain medical treatment for the claimant's disabling condition if he/she is eligible under the childhood disability provision.

Keep in mind that payments may be deposited directly into an account set up for the claimant with you as payee. As soon as you set up such an account, contact us for more information about receiving the claimant's payments using direct deposit.

Form **SSA-11-BK** (01-2014) EF (01-2014) Page 7

A REMINDER TO PAYEE APPLICANTS

TELEPHONE NUMBER(S) TO CALL IF YOU HAVE A QUESTION OR SOMETHING TO REPORT	BEFORE YOU RECEIVE A DECISION NOTICE	SSA OFFICE	DATE REQUEST RECEIVED
	AFTER YOU RECEIVE A DECISION NOTICE		

RECEIPT FOR YOUR REQUEST

Your request for SSI payments on behalf of the individual(s) named below has been received and will be processed as quickly as possible.

You should hear from us within______days after you have given us all the information we requested. Some claims may take longer if additional information is needed.

In the meantime, if you change your address, or if there is some other change that may affect the benefits payable, you - or someone for you - should report the change. The changes to be reported are listed on the reverse.

Always give us the claim number of the beneficiary when writing or telephoning about the claim.

If you have any questions about this application, we will be glad to help you.

BENEFICIARY	SOCIAL SECURITY CLAIM NUMBER

Privacy Act Statement - Collection and Use of Personal Information

Sections 205(a) and 205(j) of the Social Security Act, as amended, authorize us to collect this information. We will use the information you provide to determine if you are qualified to serve as a representative payee. Furnishing us this information is voluntary. However, failing to provide all or part of the information could prevent us from making a determination to select you as a representative payee.

We rarely use the information you supply for any purpose other than for determining continuing eligibility. However, we may use it for the administration and integrity of our programs. We may also disclose information to another person or to another agency in accordance with approved routine uses, which include but are not limited to the following: 1. To enable a third party or an agency to assist us in establishing rights to our benefits and coverage; 2. To comply with Federal laws requiring the release of information from our records (e.g., to the Government Accountability Office and Department of Veterans Affairs); 3. To make determinations for eligibility in similar health and income maintenance programs at the Federal, State, and local level; and, 4. To facilitate statistical research, audit, or investigative activities necessary to assure the integrity and improvement of our programs. (e.g., to the Bureau of Census and to private entities under contract with us).

We may also use the information you provide in computer matching programs. Matching programs compare our records with records kept by other Federal, State, or local government agencies. We use the information from these matching programs to establish or verify a person's eligibility for federally funded or administered benefit programs and for repayment of incorrect payments or delinquent debts under these programs.

A complete list of routine uses for this information is available in our Privacy Act Systems of Records Notice entitled, Master Representative Payee File, 60-0222. Additional information regarding these and other systems of records notices are available on-line at www.socialsecurity.gov or at your local Social Security office.

Paperwork Reduction Act Statement - This information collection meets the requirements of 44 U.S.C. § 3507, as amended by section 2 of the Paperwork Reduction Act of 1995. You do not need to answer these questions unless we display a valid Office of Management and Budget (OMB) control number. We estimate that it will take about 11 minutes to read the instructions, gather the facts, and answer the questions. ***Send only comments relating to our time estimate above to***: *SSA, 6401 Security Blvd, Baltimore, MD 21235-0001.*

SPECIAL BENEFITS FOR WORLD WAR II VETERANS
Information for Representative Payees Who Receive Special Benefits for WW II Veterans

YOU MUST NOTIFY THE SOCIAL SECURITY ADMINISTRATION PROMPTLY IF ANY OF THE FOLLOWING EVENTS OCCUR AND PROMPTLY RETURN ANY PAYMENT TO WHICH THE CLAIMANT IS NOT ENTITLED:

- the claimant DIES (special veterans entitlement ends the month after the claimant dies);
- the claimant returns to the United States for a calendar month or longer;
- the claimant moves or changes the place where he/she actually lives;
- the claimant receives a pension, annuity or other recurring payment (includes workers' compensation, veterans benefits or disability benefits), or the amount of the annuity changes;
- the claimant is or has been deported or removed from U.S.;
- the claimant has an UNSATISFIED FELONY WARRANT (or in jurisdictions that do not define crimes as felonies, a crime punishable by death or imprisonment exceeding 1 year) issued for his/her arrest;
- the claimant is violating a condition of probation or parole under State or Federal law.

In addition to these events about the claimant, you must also notify us if:

- YOU change your address;
- YOU are convicted of a felony or any offense under State or Federal law which results in imprisonment for more than 1 year;
- YOU have an UNSATISFIED FELONY WARRANT (or in jurisdictions that do not define crimes as felonies, a crime punishable by death or imprisonment exceeding 1 year) issued for your arrest.

BENEFITS MAY STOP IF ANY OF THE ABOVE EVENTS OCCUR. You can make your reports by telephone, mail or in person. You can contact any U.S. Embassy, Consulate, Veterans Affairs Regional Office in the Philippines or any U.S. Social Security Office.

REMEMBER:

- payments must be used for the claimant's current needs or saved if not currently needed;
- you may be held liable for repayment of any payments not used for the claimant's needs or of any overpayment that occurred due to your fault;
- you must account for benefits when so asked by the Social Security Administration. You will keep records of how benefits were spent so you can provide us with a correct accounting;
- to let us know, as soon as you know you are unable to continue as representative payee or the claimant no longer needs a payee.

A REMINDER TO PAYEE APPLICANTS

TELEPHONE NUMBER(S) TO CALL IF YOU HAVE A QUESTION OR SOMETHING TO REPORT	BEFORE YOU RECEIVE A DECISION NOTICE	SSA OFFICE	DATE REQUEST RECEIVED
	AFTER YOU RECEIVE A DECISION NOTICE		

RECEIPT FOR YOUR REQUEST

Your request for Special benefits for WW II Veterans on behalf of the individual(s) named below has been received and will be processed as quickly as possible.

You should hear from us within______ days after you have given us all the information we requested. Some claims may take longer if additional information is needed.

In the meantime, if you change your address, or if there is some other change that may affect the benefits payable, you - or someone for you - should report the change. The changes to be reported are listed on the reverse.

Always give us the claim number of the beneficiary when writing or telephoning about the claim.

If you have any questions about this application, we will be glad to help you.

BENEFICIARY	SOCIAL SECURITY CLAIM NUMBER

Privacy Act Statement - Collection and Use of Personal Information

Sections 205(a) and 205(j) of the Social Security Act, as amended, authorize us to collect this information. We will use the information you provide to determine if you are qualified to serve as a representative payee. Furnishing us this information is voluntary. However, failing to provide all or part of the information could prevent us from making a determination to select you as a representative payee.

We rarely use the information you supply for any purpose other than for determining continuing eligibility. However, we may use it for the administration and integrity of our programs. We may also disclose information to another person or to another agency in accordance with approved routine uses, which include but are not limited to the following: 1. To enable a third party or an agency to assist us in establishing rights to our benefits and coverage; 2. To comply with Federal laws requiring the release of information from our records (e.g., to the Government Accountability Office and Department of Veterans Affairs); 3. To make determinations for eligibility in similar health and income maintenance programs at the Federal, State, and local level; and, 4. To facilitate statistical research, audit, or investigative activities necessary to assure the integrity and improvement of our programs. (e.g., to the Bureau of Census and to private entities under contract with us).

We may also use the information you provide in computer matching programs. Matching programs compare our records with records kept by other Federal, State, or local government agencies. We use the information from these matching programs to establish or verify a person's eligibility for federally funded or administered benefit programs and for repayment of incorrect payments or delinquent debts under these programs.

A complete list of routine uses for this information is available in our Privacy Act Systems of Records Notice entitled, Master Representative Payee File, 60-0222. Additional information regarding these and other systems of records notices are available on-line at www.socialsecurity.gov or at your local Social Security office.

Paperwork Reduction Act Statement - This information collection meets the requirements of 44 U.S.C. § 3507, as amended by section 2 of the Paperwork Reduction Act of 1995. You do not need to answer these questions unless we display a valid Office of Management and Budget (OMB) control number. We estimate that it will take about 11 minutes to read the instructions, gather the facts, and answer the questions. ***Send only comments relating to our time estimate above to***: *SSA, 6401 Security Blvd, Baltimore, MD 21235-0001.*

Form **SSA-11-BK** (01-2014) EF (01-2014) Page 10

FUNCTION REPORT - ADULT - Form SSA-3373-BK

READ ALL OF THIS INFORMATION BEFORE YOU BEGIN COMPLETING THIS FORM

IF YOU NEED HELP

If you need help with this form, complete as much of it as you can and call the phone number provided on the letter sent with the form, or contact the person who asked you to complete the form. If you need the address or phone number for the office that provided the form, you can get it by calling Social Security at 1-800-772-1213.

HOW TO COMPLETE THIS FORM

The information that you give us on this form will be used by the office that makes the disability decision on your disability claim. You can help them by completing as much of the form as you can.

It is important that you tell us about your activities and abilities.

- Print or type.
- **DO NOT LEAVE ANSWERS BLANK.** If you do not know the answer or the answer is "none" or "does not apply," please write "don't know" or "none" or "does not apply."
- Do not ask a doctor or hospital to complete this form.
- Be sure to explain an answer if the question asks for an explanation, or if you think you need to explain an answer.
- If more space is needed to answer any questions, use the "REMARKS" section on Page 8, and show the number of the question being answered.

REMEMBER TO GIVE US THE NAME AND ADDRESS OF THE PERSON COMPLETING THIS FORM ON PAGE 8

Privacy Act and Paperwork Reduction Act Statements

Collection and Use of Personal Information - Sections 205(a), 1631(d)(1) and 1631(e)(1) of the Social Security Act (42 U.S.C. § 404), as amended, authorize us to collect this information. We will use the information you provide to assist us in making a decision on your claim.

Furnishing us this information is voluntary. However, failing to provide us with all or part of the information could prevent us from making an accurate decision on your claim.

We rarely use the information you supply for any purpose other than the reason stated above. However, we may use it for the administration and integrity of Social Security programs. We may also disclose information to another person or to another agency in accordance with approved routine uses, which include but are not limited to the following:

1. To enable a third party or an agency to assist Social Security in establishing rights to Social Security benefits and/or coverage;
2. To comply with Federal laws requiring the release of information from Social Security records (e.g., to the Government Accountability Office and Department of Veterans' Affairs);
3. To make determinations for eligibility in similar health and income maintenance programs at the Federal, State, and local level; and,
4. To facilitate statistical research, audit, or investigative activities necessary to assure the integrity and improvement of Social Security programs (e.g., to the Bureau of the Census and private concerns under contract to Social Security).

We may also use the information you provide in computer matching programs. Matching programs compare our records with records kept by other Federal, State, or local government agencies. Information from these matching programs can be used to establish or verify a person's eligibility for federally-funded or administered benefit programs and for repayment of payments or delinquent debts under these programs.

A complete list of routine uses for this information is available in our System of Records Notices entitled, Master Files of Social Security Number (SSN) Holders and SSN Applications System, 60-0058; Claims Folders Systems, 60-0089; and Master Beneficiary Record, 60-0090. These notices, additional information regarding this form, and information regarding our systems and programs, are available on-line at www.socialsecurity.gov or at any local Social Security office.

Paperwork Reduction Act Statement - This information collection meets the requirements of 44 U.S.C. § 3507, as amended by section 2 of the Paperwork Reduction Act of 1995. You do not need to answer these questions unless we display a valid Office of Management and Budget control number. We estimate that it will take about 61 minutes to read the instructions, gather the facts, and answer the questions. **SEND OR BRING THE COMPLETED FORM TO THE OFFICE THAT REQUESTED IT. If you do not have that address, you may call Social Security at 1-800-772-1213 (TTY 1-800-325-0778).** *You may send comments on our time estimate above to:* SSA, 6401 Security Blvd., Baltimore, MD 21235-6401. ***Send only comments relating to our time estimate to this address, not the completed form.***

PLEASE REMOVE THIS SHEET BEFORE RETURNING THE COMPLETED FORM.

SOCIAL SECURITY ADMINISTRATION

Form Approved
OMB No. 0960-0681

FUNCTION REPORT - ADULT

How your illnesses, injuries, or conditions limit your activities

For SSA Use Only
Do not write in this box.

Related SSN ____________
Number Holder ____________

SECTION A - GENERAL INFORMATION

1. **NAME OF DISABLED PERSON** *(First, Middle Initial, Last)*

2. **SOCIAL SECURITY NUMBER**

3. **YOUR DAYTIME TELEPHONE NUMBER** *(If there is no telephone number where you can be reached, please give us a daytime number where we can leave a message for you.)*

______ ____________ ☐ Your Number ☐ Message Number ☐ None

Area Code *Phone Number*

4. a. Where do you live? *(Check one.)*

☐ House ☐ Apartment ☐ Boarding House ☐ Nursing Home
☐ Shelter ☐ Group Home ☐ Other *(What?)* ____________

b. With whom do you live? *(Check one.)*

☐ Alone ☐ With Family ☐ With Friends
☐ Other *(Describe relationship.)* ____________

SECTION B - INFORMATION ABOUT YOUR ILLNESSES, INJURIES, OR CONDITIONS

5. How do your illnesses, injuries, or conditions limit your ability to work?

Form **SSA-3373-BK** (01-2013) ef (01-2013) Page 1
Use (12-2009) Edition until exhausted

SECTION C - INFORMATION ABOUT DAILY ACTIVITIES

6. Describe what you do from the time you wake up until going to bed.

7. Do you take care of anyone else such as a wife/husband, children, grandchildren, parents, friend, other? ☐ Yes ☐ No

   If "YES," for whom do you care, and what do you do for them?

8. Do you take care of pets or other animals? ☐ Yes ☐ No

   If "YES," what do you do for them?

9. Does anyone help you care for other people or animals? ☐ Yes ☐ No

   If "YES," who helps, and what do they do to help?

10. What were you able to do before your illnesses, injuries, or conditions that you can't do now?

11. Do the illnesses, injuries, or conditions affect your sleep? ☐ Yes ☐ No

    If "YES," how?

12. **PERSONAL CARE** (Check here ☐ if **NO PROBLEM** with personal care.)

    a. Explain how your illnesses, injuries, or conditions affect your ability to:

    Dress

    Bathe

    Care for hair

    Shave

    Feed self

    Use the toilet

    Other

b. Do you need any special reminders to take care of personal needs and grooming? ☐ Yes ☐ No

If "YES," what type of help or reminders are needed? ______

______

c. Do you need help or reminders taking medicine? ☐ Yes ☐ No

If "YES," what kind of help do you need? ______

______

13. **MEALS**

a. Do you prepare your own meals? ☐ Yes ☐ No

If "Yes," what kind of food do you prepare? (For example, sandwiches, frozen dinners, or complete meals with several courses.) ______

______

How often do you prepare food or meals? (For example, daily, weekly, monthly.)

______

How long does it take you? ______

Any changes in cooking habits since the illness, injuries, or conditions began?

______

b. If "No," explain why you cannot or do not prepare meals. ______

______

14. **HOUSE AND YARD WORK**

a. List household chores, both indoors and outdoors, that you are able to do. (For example, cleaning, laundry, household repairs, ironing, mowing, etc.) ______

______

b. How much time does it take you, and how often do you do each of these things?

______

c. Do you need help or encouragement doing these things? ☐ Yes ☐ No

If "YES," what help is needed? ______

______

d. If you don't do house or yard work, explain why not. ______

______

15. **GETTING AROUND**

a. How often do you go outside? ______

If you don't go out at all, explain why not. ______

______

b. When going out, how do you travel? *(Check all that apply.)*

☐ Walk ☐ Drive a car ☐ Ride in a car ☐ Ride a bicycle

☐ Use public transportation ☐ Other *(Explain)* ______

c. When going out, can you go out alone? ☐ Yes ☐ No

If "NO," explain why you can't go out alone. ______

______

d. Do you drive? ☐ Yes ☐ No

If you don't drive, explain why not. ______

______

16. **SHOPPING**

a. If you do any shopping, do you shop: *(Check all that apply.)*

☐ In stores ☐ By phone ☐ By mail ☐ By computer

b. Describe what you shop for. ______

______

c. How often do you shop and how long does it take? ______

______

17. **MONEY**

a. Are you able to:

Pay bills	☐ Yes	☐ No	Handle a savings account	☐ Yes	☐ No
Count change	☐ Yes	☐ No	Use a checkbook/money orders	☐ Yes	☐ No

Explain all "NO" answers. ______

______

b. Has your ability to handle money changed since the illnesses, injuries, or conditions began? ☐Yes ☐No

If "YES," explain how the ability to handle money has changed. ______________________

____

18. **HOBBIES AND INTERESTS**

a. What are your hobbies and interests? (For example, reading, watching TV, sewing, playing sports, etc.)

____

____

b. How often and how well do you do these things? ______________________

____

c. Describe any changes in these activities since the illnesses, injuries, or conditions began.

____

____

19. **SOCIAL ACTIVITIES**

a. Do you spend time with others? *(In person, on the phone, on the computer, etc.)* ☐Yes ☐No

If "YES," describe the kinds of things you do with others. ______________________

____

How often do you do these things? ______________________

b. List the places you go on a regular basis. (For example, church, community center, sports events, social groups, etc.) ______________________

____

Do you need to be reminded to go places? ☐Yes ☐No

How often do you go and how much do you take part? ______________________

____

Do you need someone to accompany you? ☐Yes ☐No

c. Do you have any problems getting along with family, friends, neighbors, or others? ☐ Yes ☐ No

If "YES," explain. ______

______

d. Describe any changes in social activities since the illnesses, injuries, or conditions began.

______

______

SECTION D - INFORMATION ABOUT ABILITIES

20. a. Check any of the following items that your illnesses, injuries, or conditions affect:

☐ Lifting	☐ Walking	☐ Stair Climbing	☐ Understanding
☐ Squatting	☐ Sitting	☐ Seeing	☐ Following Instructions
☐ Bending	☐ Kneeling	☐ Memory	☐ Using Hands
☐ Standing	☐ Talking	☐ Completing Tasks	☐ Getting Along With Others
☐ Reaching	☐ Hearing	☐ Concentration	

Please explain how your illnesses, injuries, or conditions affect each of the items you checked. (For example, you can only lift [how many pounds], or you can only walk [how far])

______

______

______

b. Are you: ☐ Right Handed? ☐ Left Handed?

c. How far can you walk before needing to stop and rest? ______

If you have to rest, how long before you can resume walking? ______

______

d. For how long can you pay attention? ______

e. Do you finish what you start? *(For example, a conversation, chores, reading, watching a movie.)* ☐ Yes ☐ No

f. How well do you follow written instructions? (For example, a recipe.) ______

______

g. How well do you follow spoken instructions? ______

______

______

h. How well do you get along with authority figures? (For example, police, bosses, landlords or teachers.) ____________________

____

i. Have you ever been fired or laid off from a job because of problems getting along with other people? ☐ Yes ☐ No

If "YES," please explain. ____________________

____

If "YES," please give name of employer. ____________________

j. How well do you handle stress? ____________________

____

k. How well do you handle changes in routine? ____________________

____

l. Have you noticed any unusual behavior or fears? ☐ Yes ☐ No

If "YES," please explain. ____________________

____

21. Do you use any of the following? *(Check all that apply.)*

☐ Crutches	☐ Cane	☐ Hearing Aid
☐ Walker	☐ Brace/Splint	☐ Glasses/Contact Lenses
☐ Wheelchair	☐ Artificial Limb	☐ Artificial Voice Box

☐ Other (Explain) ____________________

Which of these were prescribed by a doctor? ____________________

____

When was it prescribed? ____________________

____

When do you need to use these aids? ____________________

____

22. Do you currently take any medicines for your illnesses, injuries, or conditions? ☐ Yes ☐ No

If "YES, "do any of your medicines cause side effects? ☐ Yes ☐ No

If "YES," please explain. (Do not list all of the medicines that you take. List only the medicines that cause side effects.)

NAME OF MEDICINE	SIDE EFFECTS YOU HAVE

SECTION E - REMARKS

Use this section for any added information you did not show in earlier parts of this form. When you are done with this section (or if you didn't have anything to add), be sure to complete the fields at the bottom of this page.

Name of person completing this form (Please print)		Date *(month, day, year)*
Address (Number and Street)	Email address (optional)	
City	State	ZIP Code

FUNCTION REPORT - ADULT - THIRD PARTY Form SSA-3380-BK

READ ALL OF THIS INFORMATION BEFORE YOU BEGIN COMPLETING THIS FORM

IF YOU NEED HELP

If you need help with this form, complete as much of it as you can and call the phone number provided on the letter sent with the form, or contact the person who asked you to complete the form. If you need the address or phone number for the office that provided the form, you can get it by calling Social Security at 1-800-772-1213 (TTY 1-800-325-0778).

HOW TO COMPLETE THIS FORM

The information that you give on this form will be used to make a decision on the disabled person's claim. You can help by completing as much of the form as you can. When a question refers to the "disabled person," it refers to the person who is applying for or receiving disability benefits.

It is important that you tell us what you know about the disabled person's activities and abilities.

DO NOT ASK THE DISABLED PERSON TO GIVE YOU ANSWERS

- Print or type.
- **DO NOT LEAVE ANSWERS BLANK.** If you do not know the answer or the answer is "none" or "does not apply," please write "don't know" or "none" or "does not apply."
- Do not ask a doctor or hospital to complete this form.
- Be sure to explain an answer if the question asks for an explanation, or if you think you need to explain an answer.
- If you need more space to answer any questions, use the "REMARKS" section on Page 8, and show the number of the question being answered.

REMEMBER TO GIVE US THE NAME AND ADDRESS OF THE PERSON COMPLETING THIS FORM ON PAGE 8

Privacy Act and Paperwork Reduction Act Statements

Sections 205(a), 1631(d)(1) and 1631(e)(1) of the Social Security Act, as amended, authorize us to collect this information. We will use this information to process the named claimant's claim.

Furnishing us the information is voluntary. However, failing to provide us with all or part of the requested information may prevent us from making an accurate and timely decision on the named claimant's claim.

We rarely use this information for any purpose other than for making a decision regarding entitlements to benefits. However, we may use it for the administration and integrity of Social Security programs. We may also disclose information to another agency in accordance with approved routine uses, which include, but are not limited to the following:

1. To enable a third party or agency to assist Social Security in establishing rights to Social Security benefits and/or coverage;

2. To comply with Federal laws requiring the release of information from our records (e.g., to the Government Accountability Office and the Department of Veterans Affairs);

3. To make determinations for eligibility in similar health and income maintenance programs at the Federal, State, and local level; and

4. To facilitate statistical research, audit, or investigatory activities necessary to assure the integrity and improvement of Social Security programs.

We may also use the information you provide in computer matching programs. Matching programs compare our records with records kept by other Federal, State, or local government agencies. Information from these matching programs can be used to establish or verify a person's eligibility for federally-funded and administered benefit programs and for repayment of payments or delinquent debts under these programs.

A complete list of routine uses of this information is available in our Privacy Act Systems of Records Notices entitled, Claims Folders Systems, 60-0089, and Electronic Disability (eDib) Claim File, 60-0320. These notices, additional information regarding our programs and systems, are available online at www.socialsecurity.gov or at any local Social Security office.

Paperwork Reduction Act Statement - This information collection meets the requirements of 44 U.S.C. §3507, as amended by Section 2 of the Paperwork Reduction Act of 1995. You do not need to answer these questions unless we display a valid Office of Management and Budget (OMB) control number. We estimate that it will take about 61 minutes to read the instructions, gather the facts, and answer the questions. ***Send only comments relating to our time estimate above to:*** *SSA, 6401 Security Blvd., Baltimore, MD 21235-6401.*

PLEASE REMOVE THIS SHEET BEFORE RETURNING THE COMPLETED FORM.

SOCIAL SECURITY ADMINISTRATION

Form Approved
OMB No. 0960-0635

FUNCTION REPORT- ADULT - THIRD PARTY

How the disabled person's illnesses, injuries, or conditions limit his/her activities

SECTION A - GENERAL INFORMATION

1. **NAME OF DISABLED PERSON** *(First, Middle, Last)*

2. **YOUR NAME** *(Person completing the form)*	3. **RELATIONSHIP** *(To disabled person)*	4 . **DATE** *(Month, Day, Year)*

5. **YOUR DAYTIME TELEPHONE NUMBER** *(If there is no telephone number where you can be reached, please give us a daytime number where we can leave a message for you.)*

( ) ______ - ______
Area Code *Phone Number*

☐ Your Number ☐ Message Number ☐ None

6. a. How long have you known the disabled person? ______

b. How much time do you spend with the disabled person and what do you do together?

______

7. a. Where does the disabled person live? *(Check one.)*

☐ House ☐ Apartment ☐ Boarding House ☐ Nursing Home

☐ Shelter ☐ Group Home ☐ Other (What?) ______

b. With whom does he/she live? *(Check one.)*

☐ Alone ☐ With Family ☐ With Friends

☐ Other (describe relationship) ______

SECTION B - INFORMATION ABOUT ILLNESSES, INJURIES, OR CONDITIONS

8. How do this person's illnesses, injuries, or conditions limit his/her ability to work?

______

______

______

SECTION C - INFORMATION ABOUT DAILY ACTIVITIES

9. Describe what the disabled person does from the time he/she wakes up until going to bed.

10. Does this person take care of anyone else such as a wife/husband, children, grandchildren, parents, friend, other? ☐ Yes ☐ No

    If "YES," for whom does he/she care, and what does he/she do for them?

11. Does he/she take care of pets or other animals? ☐ Yes ☐ No

    If "YES," what does he/she do for them?

12. Does anyone help this person care for other people or animals? ☐ Yes ☐ No

    If "YES," who helps, and what do they do to help?

13. What was the disabled person able to do before his/her illnesses, injuries, or conditions that he/she can't do now?

14. Do the illnesses, injuries, or conditions affect his/her sleep? ☐ Yes ☐ No

    If "YES," how?

15. **PERSONAL CARE** (Check here ☐ if **NO PROBLEM** with personal care.)

    a. Explain how the illnesses, injuries, or conditions affect this person's ability to:

    Dress

    Bathe

    Care for hair

    Shave

    Feed self

    Use the toilet

    Other

b. Does he/she need any special reminders to take care of personal needs and grooming? ☐ Yes ☐ No

If "YES," what type of help or reminders are needed? ______

c. Does he/she need help or reminders taking medicine? ☐ Yes ☐ No

If "YES," what kind of help does he/she need? ______

16. **MEALS**

a. Does the disabled person prepare his/her own meals? ☐ Yes ☐ No

If "Yes," what kind of food is prepared? (For example, sandwiches, frozen dinners, or complete meals with several courses.) ______

How often does he/she prepare food or meals? (For example, daily, weekly, monthly.)

How long does it take him/her? ______

Any changes in cooking habits since the illness, injuries, or conditions began?

b. If "No," explain why he/she cannot or does not prepare meals. ______

17. **HOUSE AND YARD WORK**

a . List household chores , both indoors and outdoors , that the disabled person is able to do .
(For example, cleaning, laundry, household repairs, ironing, mowing, etc.)

b. How much time do chores take, and how often does he/she do each of these things?

c. Does he/she need help or encouragement doing these things? ☐ Yes ☐ No

If "YES," what help is needed? ______

d. If the disabled person doesn't do house or yard work, explain why not. ______________________

____

18. **GETTING AROUND**

a. How often does this person go outside? ______________________

If he/she doesn't go out at all, explain why not. ______________________

____

b. When going out, how does he/she travel? *(Check all that apply.)*

☐ Walk ☐ Drive a car ☐ Ride in a car ☐ Ride a bicycle

☐ Use public transportation ☐ Other *(Explain)* ______________________

c. When going out, can he/she go out alone? ☐ Yes ☐ No

If "NO," explain why he/she can't go out alone. ______________________

____

d. Does the disabled person drive? ☐ Yes ☐ No

If he/she doesn't drive, explain why not. ______________________

____

____

19. **SHOPPING**

a. If the disabled person does any shopping, does he/she shop: *(Check all that apply.)*

☐ In stores ☐ By phone ☐ By mail ☐ By computer

b. Describe what he/she shops for. ______________________

____

c. How often does he/she shop and how long does it take? ______________________

____

____

20. **MONEY**

a. Is he/she able to:

Pay bills	☐ Yes	☐ No	Handle a savings account	☐ Yes	☐ No
Count change	☐ Yes	☐ No	Use a checkbook/money orders	☐ Yes	☐ No

Explain all "NO" answers. ______________________

____

b. Has the disabled person's ability to handle money changed since the illnesses, injuries, or conditions began? ☐ Yes ☐ No

If "YES," explain how the ability to handle money has changed. ______

______

______

21. **HOBBIES AND INTERESTS**

a. What are his/her hobbies and interests? (For example, reading, watching TV, sewing, playing sports, etc.) ______

______

______

b. How often and how well does he/she do these things? ______

______

______

c. Describe any changes in these activities since the illnesses, injuries, or conditions began.

______

______

______

22. **SOCIAL ACTIVITIES**

a. Does the disabled person spend time with others? *(In person, on the phone, on the computer, etc.)* ☐ Yes ☐ No

If "YES," describe the kinds of things he/she does with others. ______

______

How often does he/she do these things? ______

b. List the places he/she goes on a regular basis. (For example, church, community center, sports events, social groups, etc.) ______

______

______

Does he/she need to be reminded to go places? ☐ Yes ☐ No

How often does he/she go and how much does he/she take part? ______

______

______

Does he/she need someone to accompany him/her? ☐ Yes ☐ No

c. Does this person have any problems getting along with family, friends, neighbors, or others? ☐ Yes ☐ No

If "YES," explain. ______

d. Describe any changes in social activities since the illnesses, injuries, or conditions began.

______

SECTION D - INFORMATION ABOUT ABILITIES

23. a. Check any of the following items the disabled person's illnesses, injuries, or conditions affect:

☐ Lifting	☐ Walking	☐ Stair Climbing	☐ Understanding
☐ Squatting	☐ Sitting	☐ Seeing	☐ Following Instructions
☐ Bending	☐ Kneeling	☐ Memory	☐ Using Hands
☐ Standing	☐ Talking	☐ Completing Tasks	☐ Getting Along with Others
☐ Reaching	☐ Hearing	☐ Concentration	

Please explain how his/her illnesses, injuries, or conditions affect each of the items you checked. (For example, he/she can only lift [how many pounds], or he/she can only walk [how far])

______

b. Is the disabled person: ☐ Right Handed? ☐ Left Handed?

c. How far can he/she walk before needing to stop and rest? ______

If he/she has to rest, how long before he/she can resume walking? ______

d. For how long can the disabled person pay attention? ______

e. Does the disabled person finish what he/she starts? (For example, a conversation, chores, reading, watching a movie.) ☐ Yes ☐ No

f. How well does the disabled person follow written instructions? (For example, a recipe.)

______

g. How well does the disabled person follow spoken instructions? ______

h. How well does the disabled person get along with authority figures? (For example, police, bosses, landlords or teachers.) ______________________

____

i. Has he/she ever been fired or laid off from a job because of problems getting along with other people? ☐ Yes ☐ No

If "YES," please explain. ______________________

____

If "YES," please give name of employer. ______________________

j . How well does the disabled person handle stress? ______________________

____

____

k. How well does he/she handle changes in routine? ______________________

____

l. Have you noticed any unusual behavior or fears in the disabled person? ☐ Yes ☐ No

If "YES," please explain. ______________________

____

____

24. Does the disabled person use any of the following? *(Check all that apply.)*

☐ Crutches	☐ Cane	☐ Hearing Aid
☐ Walker	☐ Brace/Splint	☐ Glasses/Contact Lenses
☐ Wheelchair	☐ Artificial Limb	☐ Artificial Voice Box

☐ Other (*Explain*) ______________________

Which of these were prescribed by a doctor? ______________________

____

When was it prescribed? ______________________

____

When does this person need to use these aids? ______________________

____

25. Does the disabled person currently take any medicines for his/her illnesses, injuries, or conditions? ☐ Yes ☐ No

If " YES," do any of the medicines cause side effects? ☐ Yes ☐ No

If "YES," please explain. (Do not list all of the medicines that the disabled person takes. List only the medicines that cause side effects for the disabled person.)

NAME OF MEDICINE	SIDE EFFECTS PERSON HAS

SECTION E - REMARKS

Use this section for any added information you did not show in earlier parts of this form. When you are done with this section (or if you didn't have anything to add), be sure to complete the fields at the bottom of this page.

Name of person completing this form (Please print)		Date *(month, day, year)*
Address (Number and Street)	Email address (optional)	
City	State	Zip Code

Form Approved
OMB No. 3206-0140

United States
Office of Personnel Management
Retirement Operations
Boyers, PA 16017

Information Necessary for a Competency Determination

An **original** or a **certified copy** of a court order appointing a guardian or fiduciary to handle the affairs of the individual should be submitted so that the Office of Personnel Management can determine whether the applicant is or was mentally incompetent or otherwise unable to handle his or her financial or other affairs. Uncertified photocopies are not acceptable. The court order should cover the entire period of time which is in question for this determination and should address whether the alleged incompetency occurred in the past or is currently present.

If no guardian or fiduciary is appointed by a court, please provide the information described in **both** A and B below.

A. A statement from the physician who has been treating the individual. (The individual or his representative is responsible for any cost incurred in obtaining this documentation.) The physician's statement should cover, but not be limited to, the time period in question for this competency determination and should address whether the alleged incompetency occurred in the past or is currently present. The physician should provide, on his or her letterhead stationery, the information listed below. **Please provide a copy of this form to the physician.**

- History of the specific medical condition(s) which caused the individual to be incompetent, including symptoms, physical findings, results of laboratory studies, and therapy (together with the response to therapy). Please provide copies of all reports of laboratory studies, in the case of psychiatric disorders, the findings of mental status examinations and copies of all psychological test reports, and copies of all discharge summaries of hospitalizations and operative reports.
- The diagnosis should be in accordance with ICD terminology or, in the case of psychiatric disorders, with DSM IV criteria.
- The duration of the medical condition(s), including the date the condition caused incompetency and the date or expected date of full or partial recovery.

B. Affidavits from at least two persons who know the facts concerning the individual's competency, preferably one from a member of the individual's immediate family and one from a non-family member. The persons making the affidavits should state:

- The relationship to, and amount of contact with, the individual during the relevant time period.
- What actions or incidents were personally observed which would show whether the individual's condition interfered with the ability to handle personal affairs, and how often these were observed.
- The reason why a guardian or fiduciary was not appointed by the court to handle the affairs of the individual.
- Who has been handling the individual's affairs.

(Affidavits must be sworn to or affirmed before a notary public or other officer who is authorized by law to administer oaths.)

Send the documents to the above address. Be sure to include the claim number shown at the top of form RI 20-7, Representative Payee Application, with this correspondence.

Warning

Affidavits and other evidence are subject to verification by personal investigation. Any intentionally false statement, willful concealment of a material fact, or use of a writing or document knowing the same to contain a false, fictitious, or fraudulent statement or entry is a violation of the law punishable by a fine of not more than $10,000 or imprisonment of not more than 5 years, or both. (18 U.S.C. 1001)

Public Burden Statement

We estimate providing this information takes an average 60 minutes per response, including the time for reviewing instructions, getting the needed data, and reviewing the requested information. Send comments regarding our estimate or any other aspect of this form, including suggestions for reducing time needed, to the Office of Personnel Management (OPM) Retirement Services Publications Team (3206-0140), Washington, D.C. 20415-3430. The OMB Number 3206-0140 is currently valid. OPM may not collect this information, and you are not required to respond, unless this number is displayed.

Previous edition is usable

RI 30-3
Revised June 2013

United States
Office of Personnel Management
Retirement Operations
P.O. Box 45
Boyers, PA 16017-0045

Form Approved:
OMB No. 3206-0140

Date of this letter
File reference
Name of annuitant
Claim number

Representative Payee Application

The Office of Personnel Management (OPM) has received information indicating that the above-named annuitant may not be capable of handling his or her benefits under the Civil Service Retirement System or the Federal Employees Retirement System. (Note: The annuitant may be a minor child without a parent to handle the benefits.) If the annuitant cannot handle the benefits, we require that the payments be made to a court-appointed fiduciary or to a person we select to represent the annuitant. A fiduciary is a person or institution appointed by a State court to be responsible for managing funds on behalf of another person.

Under the retirement law, the preferred payee in this type of case is a court-appointed fiduciary. However, if a fiduciary has not been appointed, we have authority to make payments to a representative who is willing to act on behalf of the annuitant. In addition to receiving annuity payments, the person representing the annuitant is responsible for acting in the annuitant's best interests by using the payments to benefit the annuitant, authorizing the correct withholding of Federal income tax from the annuity, and selecting the Federally sponsored health benefits coverage for the annuitant when applicable.

Payments are made to a court-appointed fiduciary or OPM-selected representative with the clear understanding that the funds will be used or conserved for the benefit of the annuitant. In the event that part or all of the annuitant's monthly payment is not required to meet his or her current needs, the representative is required to conserve the unused amount for the annuitant's future needs. The representative will be held accountable for the funds and will have to provide written reports as OPM may require to show that the payments are being properly used for the annuitant. Further, the representative is obligated to notify OPM immediately when he or she is no longer acting for the annuitant. The representative will be held liable for any payments which may be received after the annuitant dies. Such payments must be immediately returned to the U.S. Treasury Department.

OPM will not make a payee change based on a power of attorney or the existence of a joint account with the annuitant at a financial institution. We require either a State court appointment of a fiduciary or an OPM-administered agreement before we will allow anyone other than the annuitant to receive payments or authorize actions based on this claim.

If there is a court-appointed fiduciary, he or she may apply to become payee by sending us an original or a certified copy of the court appointment in the enclosed envelope with the attached application for selection. *(Uncertified photocopies are not acceptable.)*

If there is no court-appointed fiduciary or if there is one, but you believe that you should receive the payments instead, please assist us in selecting a payee by completing the attached application and ***returning it in the enclosed envelope or to the address shown above***.

For more information, call the Retirement Information Office at 1-888-767-6738, Monday through Friday between 7:30 a.m. and 7:45 p.m. Eastern time or write to us at the address shown above. Thank you for your cooperation.

Signature

Retirement Operations

☐ If this box is checked, you must submit the information described on the enclosed form along with this application.

Enclosure: RI 30-3, *Information Necessary for a Competency Determination*

Application For Selection As Representative Payee of an Annuitant

The Office of Personnel Management is interested in selecting the most suitable person to be the payee. It is necessary, therefore, to determine your relationship to the annuitant and the extent of your ability to take care of him or her. Please make sure that you answer ***all*** of the following questions so that we can proceed as soon as possible. Court-appointed fiduciaries must send OPM an original or a certified copy of the court appointment along with this application. *(Uncertified photocopies are not acceptable.)*

Answer completely. Give explanations where required. Attach additional sheet if necessary.

Part A - Identifying Information

1. Annuitant's claim number	5. Your name and mailing address	
2. Name of annuitant		
3. Where does the annuitant live? *(Street, city, state & ZIP code)*	6. Other names you have used	
4. Your relationship to the annuitant *(For example: spouse, daughter, friend)*	7. Your social security number	8. Your date of birth *(mm/dd/yyyy)*

Part B - Information About How You Will Discharge Your Duties as Payee

	Yes	No
9. Do you live within commuting distance of the annuitant? *(If "no," explain in the Remarks section how you will take care of the annuitant's financial affairs.)*		
10. Are you currently employed? *(If "yes," show occupation here* ➔ *(If "no," explain in the Remarks section. For example, are you retired, unemployed, etc.?)*		
11. Do you have any prior experience as a representative payee? *(If "yes," explain in the Remarks section.)*		
12. Have you ever been dismissed as a representative payee or convicted of a crime related to misuse of funds? *(If "yes," explain in the Remarks section.)*		
13. Have you assumed the responsibility for providing care for the annuitant? *(If your answer is no, show in the Remarks section the name and address of the person who has assumed this responsibility.)*		
14. Have you assumed the responsibility for the annuitant's routine expenses? *(If your answer is no, show in the Remarks section the name and address of the person who has assumed these responsibilities.)*		
15. If the annuitant is not a minor, has the annuitant been adjudged incompetent by a State court? *(If your answer is yes, you must attach an original or a certified copy of the court's order or decree. Uncertified photocopies are not acceptable. If the answer is no, you must attach medical documentation showing incompetence, as described on the* ***enclosed*** *RI 30-3.)*		
16. To your knowledge, has any individual been appointed, or applied for appointment, by a State court as guardian or other fiduciary charged with responsibility for the minor's or incompetent's person and/or estate? *(If the answer is yes, you must provide us with that other person's name and address, in the Remarks section, and explain why you believe that it would be more in the interest of the annuitant that payment be made to you.)*		

17. Explain below how, if you are selected representative payee, you will use the annuity payments to meet the needs and provide for the well-being of the annuitant. If and when the annuity payments are not required to meet the current needs and provide for the well-being of the annuitant, how will you otherwise expend or conserve such monies?

Complete Part C on the other side of this page.

RI 20-7
Revised June 2013

Remarks

Part C - Certification

I certify that the above information is correct. I hereby affirm that I will comply with the following requirements if I am selected as the representative payee for the annuitant.

(1) I agree to ***promptly*** notify the Office of Personnel Management in writing when I can no longer act in the best interest of the annuitant named.

(2) I agree to ***promptly*** submit such written accountability reports as the Office of Personnel Management may require.

(3) I agree to ***promptly*** notify the Office of Personnel Management if the annuitant or I move from the addresses I furnished in Part A.

(4) I agree to ***promptly*** notify the Office of Personnel Management if the annuitant recovers the capacity to handle his or her own affairs.

(5) I agree to ***promptly*** notify the Office of Personnel Management in writing if the annuitant dies and to provide a copy of the death certificate.

(6) I agree to ***promptly*** notify the Office of Personnel Management if a disabled child marries or becomes self-supporting.

(7) I agree that I will be liable for any payments which I receive after the annuitant's death. I understand that all such payments will be considered debts to the U.S. Government and are to be immediately returned to the U.S. Treasury Department. I further understand that failure to return such payments will result in appropriate debt collection activity, including the addition of interest and administrative charges, report to collection agencies, etc.

Warning: Any intentionally false statement, willful concealment of a material fact, or use of a document knowing the same to contain false, fictitious, or fraudulent statements or entry is a violation of the law punishable by a fine of not more than $10,000 or imprisonment of not more than 5 years or both (18 U.S.C. 1001).

Signature	Telephone Number ( )	Date
	Email Address	

Privacy Act Statement

Title 5, U.S. Code, Sections 8345 and 8466, authorize solicitation of this information to determine if you will be selected as payee for the annuitant. This information may be shared and is subject to verification via paper, electronic media, or through the use of computer matching programs, with national, state, local, or other charitable or social security administrative agencies to determine and issue benefits under their programs, to obtain information necessary for determination or continuation of benefits under this program, or to report income for tax purposes. It may also be shared and verified, as noted above, with law enforcement agencies when they are investigating a violation or potential violation of civil or criminal law. Executive Order 9397 (November 22, 1943) authorizes the use of the Social Security Number to distinguish you from people with similar names. Provision of this information is voluntary; failure to supply all of the requested information may result in not selecting you as payee for the annuitant.

Public Burden Statement

We estimate this form takes an average of 30 minutes per response to complete, including the time for reviewing instructions, getting the needed data, and reviewing the completed form. Send comments regarding our estimate or any other aspect of this form, including suggestions for reducing completion time, to the Office of Personnel Management (OPM), Retirement Services Publications Team (3206-0140), Washington, D.C. 20415-3430. The OMB Number 3206-0140 is currently valid. OPM may not collect this information, and you are not required to respond, unless this number is displayed.

Reverse of RI 20-7
Revised June 2013

Service Canada

PROTECTED B (when completed)

Personal Information Banks
ESDC PPU 116, 146

Certificate of Incapability

Information about the Old Age Security and/or Canada Pension Plan beneficiary

Beneficiary's Social Insurance Number

◯ Mr. ◯ Mrs. ◯ Ms ◯ Miss Usual First Name and Initial	Last Name	
Address - No., Street, Apt., P.O. Box, R.R. and City	Province or Territory	
	Country - If other than Canada	Postal Code

Note: If you are applying on behalf of an individual who is homeless or at imminent risk of being homeless please enter the community where the individual resides.

Please note that, to be considered incapable of managing his/her own affairs, a person must be suffering from severe mental impairment or a physical illness or impairment. (Please refer to the questions below.) If you are related by blood or marriage to the incapable individual or to the person applying to administer the benefits of the incapable individual, you cannot certify the individual's incapability.

Does the person named above have:

1. Good **general knowledge** of what is happening to his/her money or investments?	◯ Yes ◯ No	Comments
2. Sufficient **understanding** of the concept of time, in order to pay bills promptly?	◯ Yes ◯ No	Comments
3. Sufficient **memory** to keep track of financial transactions and decisions?	◯ Yes ◯ No	Comments
4. Ability to **balance** accounts and bills?	◯ Yes ◯ No	Comments
5. Significant **impairment of judgement** due to altered intellectual function?	◯ Yes ◯ No	Comments

In addition:

6A. How long have you known this person?	**6B.** Please state this person's date of birth.
7. Do you consider this person **capable** of managing his/her own affairs? ◯ Yes ◯ No	**If no**, is improvement expected? (Provide date)

Complete questions 8 and 9 if you are a medical professional (Physician, Registered Nurse, Nurse Practitioner, Psychologist, or Psychiatrist).

8. Diagnosis of impairment	Date impairment started
9. Comments	

Service Canada delivers Employment and Social Development Canada programs and services for the Government of Canada.

SC ISP-3505 (2015-01-15) E 1 of 2 Disponible en français Canada

PROTECTED B (when completed)

Beneficiary's Social Insurance Number

Complete questions 10 and 11 if you are a designated non-medical professional (social worker, lawyer or clergyman).

10. Description of impairment	Date impairment started
11. Comments	

To be completed by both medical and designated non-medical professionals, if certifying the incapability of a senior who is homeless or at imminent risk of being homeless.

12. Please complete the following certification:

I am a member in good standing of ______________________________

(Name of Professional Association / Organization)

Membership/Registration Number: ______________________________

Note: If you make a false or misleading statement, you may be subject to an administrative monetary penalty and interest, if any, under the *Canada Pension Plan* or the *Old Age Security Act*, or may be charged with an offence. Any benefits you received or obtained to which there was no entitlement would have to be repaid.

Name and signature of designated individual (medical professional, social worker, lawyer, or clergyman) completing this form.

First Name and Initial	Last Name	Signature **X**		Date
Address - No., Street, Apt., P.O. Box, R.R. and City		Province or Territory		Telephone
		Country	Postal Code	Profession

FOR OFFICE USE ONLY

Approval	Reason for Disapproval	Reassessment Date	Signature	Date
◯ Yes ◯ No				

Service
Canada

Service Canada Offices

Old Age Security

Mail your forms to:
The nearest Service Canada office listed below.
From outside of Canada: The Service Canada office in the **province where you last resided**.

Need help completing the forms?
Canada or the United States: **1-800-277-9914**
All other countries: **613-990-2244** (we accept collect calls)
TTY: **1-800-255-4786**
Important: Please have your social insurance number ready when you call.

NEWFOUNDLAND AND LABRADOR
Service Canada
PO Box 9430 Station A
St. John's NL A1A 2Y5
CANADA

PRINCE EDWARD ISLAND
Service Canada
PO Box 8000 Station Central
Charlottetown PE C1A 8K1
CANADA

NOVA SCOTIA
Service Canada
PO Box 1687 Station Central
Halifax NS B3J 3J4
CANADA

NEW BRUNSWICK
Service Canada
PO Box 250 Station A
Fredericton NB E3B 4Z6
CANADA

QUEBEC
Service Canada
PO Box 1816 Station Terminus
Quebec QC G1K 7L5
CANADA

ONTARIO
For postal codes beginning with "L, M or N"
Service Canada
PO Box 5100 Station D
Scarborough ON M1R 5C8
CANADA

ONTARIO
For postal codes beginning with "K or P"
Service Canada
PO Box 2013 Station Main
Timmins ON P4N 8C8
CANADA

MANITOBA AND SASKATCHEWAN
Service Canada
PO Box 818 Station Main
Winnipeg MB R3C 2N4
CANADA

ALBERTA / NORTHWEST TERRITORIES AND NUNAVUT
Service Canada
PO Box 2710 Station Main
Edmonton AB T5J 2G4
CANADA

BRITISH COLUMBIA AND YUKON
Service Canada
PO Box 1177 Station CSC
Victoria BC V8W 2V2
CANADA

Disponible en français

SC ISP-3501-OAS (2014-01-24) E

Canada

Service
Canada

PROTECTED B (when completed)
Personal Information Banks
ESDC PPU 116, 146 and 175

Agreement to administer benefits under the Old Age Security Act and/or the Canada Pension Plan by a Private Trustee

Trustees must maintain yearly records of the monies received and spent for our beneficiaries. Should the Minister want an accounting report, the trustee must provide the requested documentation for the applicable year(s).

It is very important that you:

- use a **pen** and **print** as clearly as possible.

Beneficiary's Social Insurance Number

The information contained on this form is essential for payments of benefits under the *Old Age Security Act* and/or the *Canada Pension Plan* to persons acting on behalf of a beneficiary who is incapable of managing his/her own affairs. It is retained in the information bank relating to the benefit being paid. Under the *Privacy Act*, the beneficiary has the right to request a copy of this record.

Old Age Security and/or Canada Pension Plan beneficiary

◯ Mr. ◯ Mrs. ◯ Ms. ◯ Miss Usual First Name and Initial	Last Name	
Home Address - No., Street, Apt., P.O. Box, R.R. and City	Province or Territory	
	Country - If other than Canada	Postal Code

I, the undersigned, agree to receive benefits under the *Old Age Security Act* and/or the *Canada Pension Plan* payable to the beneficiary named above and undertake, following the relevant provisions and Regulations, without charge:

1. to act on behalf of the beneficiary and, in accordance with any directions, from Employment and Social Development Canada, to administer and expend the benefits in his/her best interests;
2. to complete an accounting report for all benefits received and the payments made from them, upon request from Employment and Social Development Canada;
3. to notify Employment and Social Development Canada if the beneficiary changes address, becomes absent from Canada, dies, ceases to be incapable of managing his/her own affairs or if the trusteeship ends. And to provide any other information or evidence, and to do anything that the *Old Age Security Act* and/or the *Canada Pension Plan* or their Regulations would require from the beneficiary; and
4. to return uncashed, if the beneficiary should die, all his/her *Old Age Security* and/or *Canada Pension Plan* benefit payments which remain uncashed at the time of his/her death or which may be issued after the month of death, and to reimburse Her Majesty the Queen in Right of Canada for any loss sustained by her through the cashing of such payments.

NOTE: If you make a false or misleading statement, you may be subject to an administrative monetary penalty and interest, if any, under the *Canada Pension Plan* or the *Old Age Security Act*, or may be charged with an offence. Any benefits you received or obtained to which there was no entitlement would have to be repaid.

IN WITNESS WHEREOF, I execute this document under seal this ______ day of ____________ of the year ________ .

X ______ **Signature of Trustee**			**Signed, Sealed and Delivered in the presence of** X ______ **Signature of Witness**		
Name of Trustee - Please print			Name of Witness - Please print		
Address of Trustee - No., St., Apt., P.O. Box, R.R.			Address of Witness - No., St., Apt., P.O. Box, R.R.		
City, Town or Village		Province or Territory	City, Town or Village		Province or Territory
Country	Postal Code	Telephone number	Country	Postal Code	Telephone number
Relationship, if any, to the Beneficiary			Occupation of Witness		

Service Canada delivers Employment and Social Development Canada programs and services for the Government of Canada.

SC ISP-3506 (2014-01-01) E

Disponible en français

Canada

Service Canada

PROTECTED B (when completed)

Personal Information Banks
ESDC PPU 116, 146

Agreement to administer benefits under the Old Age Security Act and/or the Canada Pension Plan by an Agency or Institution

Trustees must maintain yearly records of the monies received and spent for our beneficiaries. Should the Minister want an accounting report, the trustee must provide the requested documentation for the applicable year(s).

Beneficiary's Social Insurance Number

It is very important that you:
- use a **pen** and **print** as clearly as possible.

The information contained on this form is essential for payments of benefits under the *Old Age Security Act* and/or the *Canada Pension Plan* to persons acting on behalf of a beneficiary who is incapable of managing his/her own affairs. It is retained in the information bank relating to the benefit being paid. Under the *Privacy Act*, the beneficiary has the right to request a copy of this record.

Old Age Security and/or Canada Pension Plan beneficiary

○ Mr. ○ Mrs. ○ Ms. ○ Miss	Usual First Name and Initial	Last Name

Agency or Institution

Official Name of Agency or Institution		
Address - No., Street, Apt., P.O. Box, R.R. and City	Province or Territory	
	Country - If other than Canada	Postal Code

We hereby agree, where so appointed, to receive benefits payable to any beneficiary under the *Old Age Security Act* and/or the *Canada Pension Plan* that Employment and Social Development Canada may direct to be paid to this agency or institution, and undertake without charge:

1. to act on behalf of the beneficiary, and, in accordance with any directions from Employment and Social Development Canada, to administer and expend the benefits in the best interests of that beneficiary;
2. to complete an accounting report for all benefits received and the payments made from them, upon request from Employment and Social Development Canada;
3. to notify Employment and Social Development Canada if the beneficiary changes address, becomes absent from Canada, dies or ceases to be incapable of managing his/her own affairs, or if the trusteeship ends; and to provide any other information or evidence, and to do anything that the *Old Age Security Act* and/or the *Canada Pension Plan* or the Regulations would require from the beneficiary; and
4. to return, if the beneficiary should die, all his/her Old Age Security and/or Canada Pension Plan benefit payments which may be made after the month of death, and to reimburse Her Majesty the Queen in Right of Canada for any loss sustained by her through the receipt of such payments.

If you are a municipality or a charitable or non-profit organization applying to administer the benefits of an incapable senior who is homeless or at imminent risk of being homeless, please complete questions 1 to 3.

Information about the individual's living situation

1. **I hereby attest that I have assessed the individual's living situation and believe that the individual named above is homeless or at imminent risk of being homeless due to the following factors (check all that apply):**
   - ☐ the absence of a fixed home address
   - ☐ a regular pattern of shelter usage
   - ☐ a precarious/unsafe/inadequate housing arrangement
   - ☐ self-identification of the individual as being homeless

Service Canada delivers Employment and Social Development Canada programs and services for the Government of Canada.

Canada

PROTECTED B (when completed)

Beneficiary's Social Insurance Number

Information about your Organization

2. **Organization Type**

I hereby attest that our organization ______________________ is:
Organization Name

- [ ] **A Municipality** incorporated under the relevant Provincial or Territorial Act (Please provide the name and section of the relevant Act) ______________________
- [ ] **A Registered Charity** (Please provide your Charitable Registration Number) ______________________
- [ ] **A Non-Profit Organization** (Please indicate if your organization possesses an exemption under the *Income Tax Act*
  - [ ] Yes *If yes, please provide proof of the exemption. If this is not available, please provide information supporting your status as a non-profit organization
  - [ ] No

3. **Please confirm that you have the relevant professional liability insurance or, in the case of municipalities, the ability to fund a liability.**

- [ ] Yes
- [ ] No

NOTE: If you make a false or misleading statement, you may be subject to an administrative monetary penalty and interest, if any, under the *Canada Pension Plan* or the *Old Age Security Act*, or may be charged with an offence. Any benefits you received or obtained to which there was no entitlement would have to be repaid.

IN WITNESS WHEREOF, this document has been executed under seal on behalf of the agency or institution named above, by its officers duly authorized in that regard, this _______ day of ________________ of the year ________ .

Signature of Representative of Agency or Institution	Signed, Sealed and Delivered in the presence of
X ______________________ Signature of Representative	X ______________________ Signature of Witness
	Name of Witness - Please print
Name of representative - Please print	Address of Witness - No., Street, Apt., P.O. Box, R.R.
Please indicate your Title	City, Town or Village / Province or Territory
	Country - if other than Canada / Postal Code / Telephone number
Telephone number	Occupation of Witness

Appendix D

Biographical Sketches of Committee Members

Paul S. Appelbaum, M.D. (*Chair*), is Elizabeth K. Dollard professor of psychiatry, medicine, and law and director of the Division of Psychiatry, Law, and Ethics in the Department of Psychiatry at the Columbia University College of Physicians and Surgeons. He is a research psychiatrist at the New York State Psychiatric Institute and an affiliated faculty member at Columbia Law School. He directs Columbia's Center for Research on Ethical, Legal, and Social Implications of Psychiatric, Neurologic, and Behavioral Genetics, and heads the Clinical Research Ethics Core for Columbia's Clinical and Translational Science Award program. Dr. Appelbaum is the author of many articles and books on law and ethics in clinical practice and research, including four that were awarded the Manfred S. Guttmacher Award from the American Psychiatric Association (APA) and the American Academy of Psychiatry and the Law. He is past president of the APA and of the American Academy of Psychiatry and the Law. He has twice served as chair of the APA Council on Psychiatry and Law and of the APA Committee on Judicial Action, and he currently chairs the APA's *Diagnostic and Statistical Manual of Mental Disorders* Steering Committee. He was a member of the MacArthur Foundation Research Networks on Mental Health and the Law and on Mandatory Outpatient Treatment and is a network scholar for the Network on Neuroscience and Law. Dr. Appelbaum has received the APA's Isaac Ray Award for "outstanding contributions to forensic psychiatry and the psychiatric aspects of jurisprudence," was Fritz Redlich fellow at the Center for Advanced Study in the Behavioral Sciences, and has been elected to the National Academy of Medicine. He performs forensic evaluations in civil and criminal cases and treats patients with a broad variety of problems.

Dr. Appelbaum is a graduate of Columbia College, received his M.D. from Harvard Medical School, and completed his residency in psychiatry at the Massachusetts Mental Health Center/Harvard Medical School in Boston.

Karen E. Anderson, M.D., M.P.H., is an associate professor of psychiatry and neurology and director of the Huntington's Disease Care, Education and Research Center at MedStar Georgetown University Hospital. She sees adult patients and families dealing with behavioral symptoms caused by neurological conditions such as Huntington's disease, Parkinson's disease, Alzheimer's disease, and brain injuries. Her work combines her lifelong interest in behavior with an interest in understanding how disease can affect the brain and cause behavioral symptoms. In addition to seeing patients and their families, Dr. Anderson is active in research. She is currently co-principal investigator for clinical trials studying medications for Huntington's disease and for tardive dyskinesia, a neurological disorder. She also is involved in research to develop treatment for the behavioral symptoms of Parkinson's disease, brain injury, and Alzheimer's disease. Dr. Anderson is on the executive committee of the Huntington Study Group, a collaborative organization of physicians and health care providers from around the world who are dedicated to clinical research on Huntington's disease. She received her medical degree from the University of Chicago Pritzker School of Medicine and her M.P.H. from the Columbia University Mailman School of Public Health.

María P. Aranda, Ph.D., joined the University of Southern California (USC) School of Social Work faculty in 1995 and holds a joint appointment with the USC Leonard Davis School of Gerontology. Her research and teaching interests address the interplay among chronic illness, social resources, and psychological well-being in low-income minority populations. Dr. Aranda has served as principal investigator or co-investigator on several key studies funded by and/or in collaboration with the National Institute of Mental Health, the National Cancer Institute, the National Institute on Aging, the Patient-Centered Outcomes Research Institute, Southern California-Clinical and Translational Science Institute (CTSI), the John A. Hartford Foundation/the Gerontological Society of America, the National Institute of Rehabilitation and Research, the Alzheimer's Association/Health Resources and Services Administration, the Los Angeles County Department of Mental Health, and the California Community Foundation. Overall, her research addresses psychosocial care for adult and late-life psychiatric disorders, linguistic and cultural adaptations of behavioral health services, and evidence-based interventions. Dr. Aranda has 30 years of licensed clinical experience in providing assessment and treatment services to middle-aged and older adults with comorbid medical and psychiatric illness. She has served on local and national boards and committees dedicated to the enhancement of practice, policy, research, and advocacy related to historically underrepresented minority populations. Dr. Aranda received her undergraduate degree in social work from the California State University, Los Angeles. She obtained her M.S.W., M.P.A., and Ph.D. from USC.

Nancy Bagatell, Ph.D., OTR/L, is an associate professor in the Division of Occupational Science and Occupational Therapy at the University of North Carolina at Chapel Hill and director of the Ph.D. program. Her research interests focus on adolescents and the transition to adulthood and independent living and on community participation in adults with autism spectrum disorders and other developmental disabilities. As an occupational scientist, she studies how sociocultural, contextual, and political phenomena facilitate and inhibit engagement in everyday occupation. Currently, Dr. Bagatell is an investigator on a longitudinal study of outcomes for adults with autism spectrum disorders and on a study focused on community integration of adults with cerebral palsy. Additionally, she is a member of an interdisciplinary team conducting research to support the development of a comprehensive service for adolescents with cerebral palsy and their families. She has worked clinically in mental health settings and with individuals with autism spectrum disorders and developmental disabilities across the life span in schools, homes, and the community. Dr. Bagatell served on the Autism Advisory Council for the State of Connecticut and worked extensively with the Connecticut Autism Resource Center. She holds a bachelor's degree in music performance from Indiana University and obtained both her M.A. in occupational therapy and her Ph.D. in occupational science from the University of Southern California.

Julie Birkenmaier, Ph.D., M.S.W., LCSW, is a professor at the Saint Louis University School of Social Work. Her research, publishing, and teaching are focused on financial capability and credit, social work practice, and older adults. She is the senior editor of *Financial Education and Capability: Research, Education, Policy, and Practice* (Oxford University Press, 2013) and *Educating for Social Justice: Transformative Experiential Learning* (Lyceum Books, 2011). She is co-author of *The Practice of Generalist Social Work* (3rd ed., Routledge, 2014) and *The Practicum Companion for Social Work: Integrating Class and Field Work* (3rd ed., Allyn & Bacon, 2011). Dr. Birkenmaier is a licensed clinical social worker. She received her M.S.W. from Saint Louis University and holds a Ph.D. in political science from the University of Missouri–St. Louis.

Nancy Neveloff Dubler, LL.B., is an attorney and a professor emerita of bioethics at the Albert Einstein College of Medicine. She was founder and director of the Division of Bioethics at Montefiore Medical Center. She is presently ethics consultant to the New York City Health and Hospitals Corporation and an adjunct professor at New York University Langone Medical Center, Division of Bioethics. Professor Dubler has written about end-of-life care, AIDS, geriatrics, prison and jail health care, research ethics, clinical ethics consultation, and bioethics mediation. She has consulted widely with academic medical centers and is a member of the New York State Task Force on Life and the Law and the New York State Stem Cell Ethics Research Board.

Laura B. Dunn, M.D., is director of the Geriatric Psychiatry Fellowship Training Program and professor in the Department of Psychiatry and Behavioral Sciences at Stanford University. She is board certified in psychiatry and geriatric psychiatry. She has served as secretary/treasurer and a board member of the American Association of Geriatric Psychiatry and is a member of the American College of Psychiatrists and the American Psychosocial Oncology Society. Dr. Dunn has extensive research and clinical experience in the evaluation and management of older adults with mood, anxiety, and cognitive disorders. She also has extensive research and clinical expertise in psycho-oncology. She is an internationally recognized expert in the study of ethical issues in clinical research (e.g., informed consent, decision-making capacity, and influences on research participation). Her research has examined ethical issues in psychiatric research and in clinical research more generally, with a focus on potentially vulnerable individuals. Her work has included randomized trials of novel methods for enhancing the informed consent process for research and assessments of potential participants' understanding of key aspects of research participation. Dr. Dunn has published extensively on empirical ethics issues in vulnerable populations. Her psycho-oncology research focuses on identifying patterns and predictors in the longitudinal course of psychological symptoms in cancer patients, as well as on developing and testing novel interventions for pervasive symptoms. She has served as a principal investigator, co-investigator, or consultant on many National Institutes of Health–funded and foundation-funded studies on issues in empirical ethics, geriatric psychiatry, and psycho-oncology.

Alan M. Jette, P.T., M.P.H., is director of the Health & Disabilities Research Institute and professor of health policy and management at the Boston University School of Public Health. His research interests include late-life exercise; evaluation of rehabilitation treatment outcomes; and the measurement, epidemiology, and prevention of disability. Dr. Jette is an international expert in the development and dissemination of contemporary outcome measurement instruments for evaluating health care quality and outcomes, and has published more than 200 peer-reviewed articles on these topics. He currently directs a project entitled "Use of Computer Adaptive Testing to Assist with the Social Security Work Disability Determination Process." He and his collaborators in the Department of Rehabilitation at the National Institutes of Health (NIH) Clinical Center are assisting the U.S. Social Security Administration in improving its work disability determination process by analyzing existing Social Security datasets and developing new measures to be used within the process. Currently, Dr. Jette directs the Boston Rehabilitation Outcome Measurement Center, funded by the National Center for Medical Rehabilitation Research/NIH; serves on the Executive Committee of the Boston Claude Pepper Older Americans Independence Center, funded by National Institute on Aging/NIH; and is project director of the New England Regional Spinal Cord Injury Center, funded by the National Institute on Disability and Rehabilitation Research (NIDRR). For the past 13 years, he has directed the Boston University Post-Doctoral Fellowship Program in Outcomes Research, funded by NIDRR, and from 1996 to 2004 he served as dean of Boston University's Sargent College of Health & Rehabilitation Sciences. He also has served on a number of Institute of Medicine and National Research Council study committees addressing issues in disability and rehabilitation, including the recent consensus study on the role of psychological testing in the Social Security Administration disability determination process. Dr. Jette has served as well on several international panels. In 2013, he was elected as a member of the National Academy of Medicine. He received a B.S. in physical therapy from the State University of New York at Buffalo in 1973 and an M.P.H. (1975) and a Ph.D. (1979) in public health from the University of Michigan.

David A. Loewenstein, Ph.D., is professor and director of neuropsychology in the Department of Psychiatry and Behavioral Sciences at the University of Miami School of Medicine. He formerly served as director of research for the Wien Center for Alzheimer's Disease and Memory Disorders at Mount Sinai Medical Center in Miami Beach, Florida. His research interests include the effects of exercise and cognitive training in mild cognitive impairment, cognitive testing in mild cognitive impairment and dementia, and predictors of progression from mild cognitive impairment to dementia. Dr. Loewenstein has a number of research interests centering on the early detection of early cognitive impairment in neurodegenerative and other brain disorders; the development of novel cognitive and functional measures; and the relationships among neuropsychological measures, neuroimaging, and other biomarkers of early Alzheimer's disease. He and other investigators in his laboratory have been involved in developing cognitive and functional interventions for normal elderly patients, as well as those with Alzheimer's disease and related disorders. Dr. Loewenstein is a board-certified neuropsychologist.

He received both an M.S. in psychology and a Ph.D. in clinical psychology from Florida State University.

Marc A. Norman, Ph.D., is a clinical professor of medical neuropsychology and director of the Neuropsychiatry/Epilepsy Clinical Evaluation Program at the University of California, San Diego, providing pre- and postsurgery evaluations and intracarotid amytal procedure cognitive testing. He also conducts intraoperative (awake) language testing for the epilepsy and brain tumor surgery groups and provides assessments for the heart/lung, kidney/pancreas, and liver transplant teams. Dr. Norman's general practice includes assessments for traumatic brain injury, stroke, concussion, dementia, memory disorders, multiple sclerosis, and a variety of other cognitive issues. He was elected as a fellow and is on the Board of Directors of the National Academy of Neuropsychology. He also serves on the Professional Advisory Board for the Epilepsy Foundation of America San Diego Chapter, and holds several other national positions. Dr. Norman received his Ph.D. in clinical psychology, with emphasis in neuropsychology, from Brigham Young University. He is a board-certified neuropsychologist and holds a diplomate in clinical neuropsychology from the American Board of Clinical Neuropsychology.

Eldar Shafir, Ph.D., is William Stewart Tod professor of psychology and public affairs at Princeton University and is co-founder and scientific director of ideas42, a social science research and development lab. He studies decision making, cognitive science, and behavioral economics. His recent research has focused on decision making in contexts of poverty and on the application of behavioral research to policy. He is past president of the Society for Judgment and Decision Making, a member of the Russell Sage Foundation Behavioral Economics Roundtable, and a senior fellow of the Canadian Institute for Advanced Research. Dr. Shafir was a member of President Barack Obama's Advisory Council on Financial Capability, and is currently vice-chair of the World Economic Forum's Global Agenda Council on Behaviour. He was named one of *Foreign Policy Magazine*'s 100 Leading Global Thinkers of 2013. Dr. Shafir has held visiting positions at the University of Chicago Graduate School of Business, the Kennedy School of Government, the Russell Sage Foundation, the Hebrew University Institute for Advanced Studies, Pompeu Fabra University in Barcelona, DiTella University in Buenos Aires, and Oxford University. He received his B.A. from Brown University and his Ph.D. from the Massachusetts Institute of Technology.

Kelly A. Thompson, Esq., has worked in the trusts and estates field since 1977, as both a trust banker and a trusts and estates attorney. Since 1995 her practice has focused on planning for persons with special needs. She serves as trustee, guardian, and representative payee for individuals with disabilities. She is a director of the Special Needs Alliance, a national group of attorneys serving the legal needs of individuals with a disability. She is a fellow of the American College of Trust and Estate Counsel and is regularly listed among Best Lawyers, Super Lawyers, and Washingtonian Top Lawyers. Ms. Thompson received her undergraduate degree from the University of Virginia and her juris doctor degree from the Fordham University School of Law. She is admitted to practice in the District of Columbia, New York, and Virginia.